BEING AND HEARING

Hau
BOOKS

www.haubooks.com

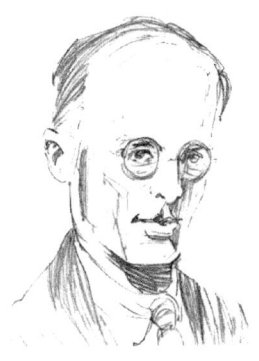

The Malinowski Monographs

In tribute to the foundational, yet productively contentious, nature of the ethnographic imagination in anthropology, this series honors the creator of the term "ethnographic theory" himself. Monographs included in this series represent unique contributions to anthropology and showcase groundbreaking work that contributes to the emergence of new ethnographically-inspired theories or challenge the way the "ethnographic" is conceived today.

BEING AND HEARING
MAKING INTELLIGIBLE WORLDS IN DEAF KATHMANDU

By Peter Graif

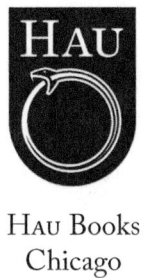

Hau Books
Chicago

Cover and layout design: Sheehan Moore

Typesetting: Prepress Plus (www.prepressplus.in)

ISBN: 978-0-9991570-3-9
LCCN: 2018943588

Hau Books
Chicago Distribution Center
11030 S. Langley
Chicago, IL 60628
www.haubooks.com

Hau Books is printed, marketed, and distributed by The University of Chicago Press.
www.press.uchicago.edu

Printed in the United States of America on acid-free paper.

For Sonya

Table of Contents

List of Figures   xi

Chapter 1. Arjun: The sense of things   1
  Homecomings   1
  Not knowing Arjun   7
  Linguistic dilemmas   16
  Making *sense*   23
  The presence of Arjun   32

Chapter 2. Intelligible worlds   37
  Necessary words   37
  Finding the deaf   46
  Deaf geographies   51
  The world is not as we think it is   61
  Raghav: being two things   68

Chapter 3. Being transparent   77
  A history of names   77
  Language as a thing seen   85
  The intelligibility of words   96

Chapter 4. Seeing politics   107
    Intelligibility play   107
    The deafness of mothers and buildings   119
    Lorem Ipsum   129
    Intelligibility replay   133

Chapter 5. Citing signs   137
    The iconic and the arbitrary . . .   137
    . . . the long and the short   141
    Deaf linguistic theory   151
    Bakery mandates   163

Chapter 6. Laxmi: The properties of people   171
    The deaf mute speaks!   171
    Being Laxmi, here and there   175
    Talk/intelligible   183
    After words   190

References   197
Acknowledgments   211
Index   213

List of Figures

Figure 1: ELEPHANT
Figure 2: WATER
Figure 3: MOUNTAIN (himal)
Figure 4: RED
Figure 5: PORTER
Figure 6: COOK
Figure 7: THINGS
Figure 8: Cover of the Nepali Sign Language Dictionary
Figure 9: HEAVY
Figure 10: IMPORTANT
Figure 11: BIG
Figure 12: COW
Figure 13: BUFFALO
Figure 14: EASY
Figure 15: CLEAR
Figure 16: DOG
Figure 17: WORK
Figure 18: Staff at the Bakery Cafe in Baneshwar, Kathmandu

All images from the Nepali Sign Language Dictionary are courtesy of the National Federation of the Deaf Nepal

CHAPTER I

Arjun: The sense of things

If there were no eternal consciousness in a man, if at the foundation of all there lay only a wildly seething power which writhing with obscure passions produced everything that is great and everything that is insignificant, if a bottomless void never satiated lay hidden beneath all—what then would life be but despair?

— Søren Kierkegaard, *Fear and Trembling*

HOMECOMINGS

Arjun Gurung is deaf. He lives in a small room on the third floor of a backpacker hotel in northeastern Nepal. His family has owned this hotel since before he was born, and over the last few years especially they've earned an international reputation as warm and capable hosts. Their hotel is located on a minor trekking route, and this location brings both tourists and tourist dollars to an otherwise remote and generally poor part of the country. Though Arjun's family has been prominent in the area for many generations, the cash generated by their hotel has allowed them to maintain this prominence over the past few decades as they, like all Nepalis, enter into increasingly global frames of reference.

I first met Arjun in the summer of 2007, when both he and I were in our late twenties. I was on a short break from fieldwork,[1] and I had booked a room in his family's hotel completely unaware that a deaf man lived there. Arjun himself had come home only recently after living for more than two decades in Kathmandu, first at a boarding school for the deaf and then later in an apartment with friends. Now back home, he stands out. In ways apparent even to outsiders, he just doesn't look like he comes from here. His family's hotel basks in a carefully maintained veneer of rural authenticity, and it is surrounded for miles on all sides by the more functional assemblage of new and old that characterizes subsistence farming. Arjun, by contrast, is instantly recognizable as an eager participant in Nepal's emerging urban middle class. He wears jeans and designer tee-shirts, he follows the international soccer scene, and he prefers foreign-brand beer to his mother's (excellent) homemade apple brandy. His habits, appearance, and disposition simply do not fit with the environment around him. By his own admission, he felt more comfortable in the city. He says he misses it dearly now that he is away.

As the only deaf person within a ten-mile walk, Arjun probably also misses the large and vibrant deaf community that comprised his daily world when he lived in Kathmandu. In Nepal, the deaf care deeply about one another. Though Arjun would no doubt laugh at the sentimentality of my words here, I think he would, with some caveats, ultimately agree. The bonds of language,

---

1.   The accounts in this book are the product of roughly four years of immersive fieldwork conducted between 2003 and 2018. In this chapter, my descriptions of Arjun draw primarily from a period about a year following our first meeting. During that time, I visited him frequently at his home, and my experiences there motivated a major shift in my methodological engagements with deaf Nepal. Previously, across a series of shorter research trips between 2003 and 2006, I focused my attention on political expression in the institutional spaces where deaf people congregate. This preliminary work anticipated the tone of my longest continuous stretch of fieldwork, which took place over eighteen months in 2007 and 2008. These years were characterized by dramatic political changes for Nepal in general and for deaf Nepal in particular. These changes culminated in a comprehensive peace agreement that ended the decades-long civil war and a contentious election that saw Nepal's first deaf politician join the country's highest legislative body (see chapter 2). During this period, I began to spend more and more time with the deaf people I knew in their mostly hearing homes, following them especially as they moved between their deaf and hearing worlds. This new approach has characterized my relationship with deaf Nepalis since then, especially in short follow-up field visits in 2009 and 2012 and in a more ongoing engagement living and working in Kathmandu from 2014 to the present.

aid, obligation, and friendship that deaf people build are frequently the most powerful and durable parts of their lives. These specifically deaf relationships often outshine (though never fully erase) all their ties to the hearing, relegating even parents, siblings, spouses, and neighbors to the emotional periphery of deaf lives. When those like Arjun from remote parts of the country arrive for the first time in deaf Kathmandu, they tend to describe the experience as a *homecoming*, steeped in feelings of kinship and belonging. For most, returning completely to the hearing world, like Arjun has done, would be unthinkable.

Arjun, however, tends to shrug off most questions about his place amongst the hearing with a characteristic reserve. He has no plans to leave, he says, so the question of whether he *likes* being back home just isn't relevant or interesting. This kind of self-effacement was very typical of Arjun in the time I knew him. He is friendly but cool, engaging but undemonstrative, and most of all always very self-composed. He tells great stories, but his affect is so flat that it can be hard to know how he intends for his audiences to react. Though I am certain that Arjun misses his deaf friends back in Kathmandu, he never admitted it to me.

Conversations about politics, however, often leave Arjun visibly angry. In particular, he is angry about rural Nepal's "lack of development," which for him seems to describe a particular mindset more than any absence of infrastructure. Nepal is a country of vast potential, he says, but it is stifled by a range of deep problems: corrupt politicians, backwards-thinking citizens, ineffective foreign aid, and—especially—an archaic and burdensome system of kinship obligations. These are familiar targets of middle-class frustration in contemporary Nepal, but for Arjun they are all explicitly rooted in a more basic question of *individual desire*. How, he would often ask, are we meant to resolve the tensions between what people want for themselves and what is good for their communities? To hear him tell it, the entirety of Nepal's recent history is a story about the rise of individualism. He attributed these transformations mostly to Western influences, though it was not always clear to me whether he understood the changes he saw as the *cause of* or the *solution to* rural Nepal's many contemporary problems. Perhaps he meant them to be both. In any case, Arjun always seemed to me preoccupied by the question of what it means to be someone who *wants* things. This same air of irresolution—where the personal and the social collide—colored every account I heard Arjun make of his life and especially his decision to return home.

Arjun is home because his parents expected him to marry and because he reluctantly agreed that it was time. He sold his few things in the capital, bought a tourist-class bus ticket to a nearby trekking hub, and walked the seven remaining hours home. Two months later, he was married. None of his friends from Kathmandu were invited to the banquet, though Arjun says he has no regrets. He says he likes being married, but he adds that he is in no rush to have children. He cites Nepal's poor political situation and a lack of good schools in the area as reasons to wait a few more years. He admits that this decision has become a point of contention with Suddha, his wife. Suddha is not deaf, nor does she know any deaf people other than her husband. She comes from a poor but well-regarded family of sharecroppers a half-day's walk from the main road. Though she is significantly better educated than her very limiting socioeconomic background would predict, her manner, disposition, and dialect nevertheless make it very clear that she was born into a household quite different from the one in which she now lives. The class dynamics at play here are nuanced, but they also boil down to some very simple facts: Arjun's maternal uncles are regional landlords of some note, and his father has a reputation for getting politicians elected; most of Suddha's male relatives, meanwhile, are day laborers.

Nevertheless, things between Arjun and Suddha moved forward quickly because everyone agreed that the marriage was such an obviously good fit. At face value, this is a strange claim. Every visible sign tells the story of the couple's very different life histories. They are affectionate with each other, but even a year after their wedding they were still often bashful and awkward in each other's company. Arjun acknowledged this tension, which he attributed to the fits and starts of their learning how to interact. But marriage negotiations have a tendency to collapse otherwise incommensurate schemes of value. Given the preference in the area for marriage between equals, it would seem that Arjun's deafness and Suddha's humble station came somehow to balance in the tally of social status that preceded their match. This is actually a very familiar type of marriage in contemporary Nepal: men with discrete, personal stigmas (e.g., various disabilities, addictions, or personality "quirks") often marry women with more gradient, familial disadvantages (e.g., low class, capital, or prestige). Though it is impolite to speak too explicitly about the benefits and compromises that a marriage alliance might bring, both families told me how relieved they are to have found each other. Even Arjun, though famously taciturn, is prone to gush about just how much he and Suddha are in love.

Despite his happy marriage, however, Arjun admits that he is desperately bored. In Kathmandu, he involved himself in political movements, dated both deaf and hearing girls, and worked as a tutor at the school that he had once attended. Then, after more than twenty years away, he came back to a "home" he had visited only a few dozen times since childhood. He spends most of his time now doing chores around the hotel, but the work is repetitive and usually better handled by his family's large and very competent staff. On top of it all, he doesn't even have other fluent signers to talk to. As Arjun puts it, there's just not a lot to do here. He enjoys managing the family's stable of horses and chatting with the international tourists who pass through town, but, these small pleasures aside, the transition has not been easy. More than once, I arrived at the hotel to find Arjun and his mother mired in the aftermath of an argument and actively ignoring each other. This is a very familiar story in contemporary Nepal's emerging middle classes: A young son from a prominent rural family is sent away to the capital city to get an education that is unavailable closer to home. While living there, he acquires tastes, habits, and ideas incompatible with the rhythms and values of everything he left behind. Though Arjun is deaf, the structure of his experience belongs to a much wider scope. He is, in many ways, very typical of an entire generation of dislocated youth.

There is a single detail, however, that makes this story unmistakably deaf: here at home, all of the people closest to Arjun believe that he is a simpleton. They think—incorrectly—that he has only a childish understanding of what goes on around him and that he is incapable of language or complex thought. They are unaware, for example, that he can read, write, and even do basic book-keeping. His English is arguably better than theirs, and he has a decent grasp of French, German, Hebrew, and Japanese. He has cultivated this polylingual-ism in a series of meticulously organized notebooks, each filled with words and phrases taught to him by his international clientele. He often studies these notebooks late into the night, and he says that one day he hopes to compile them into a universal dictionary and phrasebook. In ways that would seem ob-vious, Arjun is exceptionally intelligent. He has a bone-dry sense of humor with a strong penchant for sarcasm; he follows national politics but chooses not to vote; and he considers professional wrestling (which his parents adore) to reflect poorly on American culture. He is the only person within a half-day's walk who understands the hotel's solar electric system, and he plans to buy a few extra panels in the near future to power a television and an Xbox. Within virtually any other frame of recognition, Arjun would be unmistakable as the most cosmopolitan member of his family. Yet somehow his parents—though plainly devoted to the happiness of their only child—believe that he is an actual, literal idiot.

For reasons that are not yet clear, Arjun's family members do not easily see in him the elaborate structures of mind that they take for granted in each other and in everyone else. He is, to them, almost animal-like in his way of being a person. The precise entailments of this assessment are nuanced enough, complex enough, and culturally specific enough to justify the remainder of this chapter's attention, but as a beginning let it suffice to say that he is treated by those around him as the kind of person from whom very little should be expected and to whom very little should be offered. Neighbors and cousins talk about Arjun with diminutive pronouns more appropriate for toddlers, dogs, or bad drivers, and the trekking guides who come through town have been known to get drunk and tease him, ostensibly for not understanding that he is being teased. For her part, Arjun's mother often relates how proud she is of her son, and yet even her most boastful stories invariably highlight behaviors that would be unremarkable from any adult man seen as fully competent. That Arjun can, for example, feed and clothe himself, travel into town alone, and follow simple housekeeping routines apparently strikes her as something worth bragging about. Meanwhile, she seems not even to notice her son's many complex engagements with the world outside his home. Instead, the broader scope of Arjun's human experience—virtually everything he thinks, does, and is—remains somehow lost to the noise.

Arjun is characteristically stoic about these circumstances, but it is hard for me not to feel staggered by frustration on his behalf. After all, social life is built on the premise of intersubjectivity. Knowing other people means having ways of speculating about what they are experiencing. Skeptics might argue that we can never truly know anything about the minds of others, but in Nepal at least this posture of solipsism is at most a thought experiment and never actually a way of relating to real people in the world. Instead, under all normal circumstances, we sense purpose in the things that others do. We perceive in their actions the presence of thoughts, sentiments, and drives—unique in configuration perhaps but ultimately *human* in nature. Even when the connections between outward actions and internal mental states are hard to see, we maintain a deep trust in the fact that they exist (see Robbins 2008; Robbins and Rumsey 2008). Ethnographic research, in particular, would be inconceivable without the orienting assumption that people everywhere have minds that *make sense*. This is what Adolf Bastian famously called the "psychic unity of mankind," and it is what allows us—even in the face of stark cultural difference—to engage coherently with others. Arjun is somehow exempt from this unity at home, and in this book my aim is to understand how and why that came to be.

NOT KNOWING ARJUN

In telling Arjun's story here, my goal is not to suggest that he is in any way typical. Indeed, deaf lives in Nepal are widely diverse, and the sheer extent of Arjun's isolation is actually quite unusual. His experience of living at the margins of hearing expectations, however, is universal. Deaf lives are lived in predominantly hearing worlds, and hearing worlds often do a very poor job of relating to deaf experiences. Especially in matters of identity, language, and personhood, the deaf are constantly misunderstood. In recent years, documenting and correcting this history has been the primary aim of the newly emerging academic discipline known as deaf studies. Since its rise in the 1960s amidst the successes of humanism, feminism, and the civil rights movement, deaf studies has worked hard to demonstrate the value and complexity of everything native to deaf communities (Ladd 2003; Padden and Humphries 2009). Central to this ambition has been an explicitly ethnographic argument: namely, when we consider the various languages, beliefs, and practices of deaf communities worldwide, we should understand them not merely as adaptations to the hearing world but instead as the autonomous, constituting parts of a distinctly deaf cultural modality (see, e.g., Monaghan et al. 2003). According to this framework of analysis, Arjun's dilemma would be very familiar: though his family members see his disability, they fail completely to understand his identity.

This emphasis on identity as a driver of cultural difference has been tremendously productive for deaf studies, but there are some hard constraints on what it can reveal. It grants complexity to deaf communities precisely by stripping it from the families, publics, and contexts in which deaf people are always immersed. Arjun's mother, for example, *talks* about her son as someone flatly deprived of human capacities, but she does not always *act* as if this is so. In day-to-day practice, her engagements are much more contextually entangled. She sees Arjun affable and animated with the backpackers who pass through town, and she relies on him to attend to their needs as customers. What she seems not to perceive, however, is the substance of interiority that should normally accompany these behaviors. Even as Arjun manages food orders, guest check-ins, and complicated billing cycles effectively, she believes that he acts with no real understanding of what he does. As she puts it, "The tourists are nice to him, but he doesn't understand them. He brings them the menus, but he doesn't know why. He doesn't even know what menus are for. He smiles because they smile."

The tourists themselves, meanwhile, interpreted their interactions with Arjun very differently. They felt uncomfortable initially, they said, but ultimately they were surprised by how easy it was to interact with him despite his deafness. Indeed, Arjun is a master at putting his guests at ease. He shows interest in their lives, and he teaches them with obvious pleasure how he communicates effectively. On the occasions that I observed it, this would usually begin with simple gestures supported by notes written on scraps of paper, which then progressed over the course of the evening through increasingly elaborate acts of pantomime (accompanied, usually, by no small amount of both laughter and alcohol). People *like* Arjun. He is an excellent host. Every morning, before the tourists set off to continue further up the mountain, they linger with him over long goodbyes. His notebooks are filled with the messages of remembrance that they have left, and he regularly gets thick stacks of postcards delivered from abroad. When I asked Arjun's mother about these interactions, however, she merely smiled and reaffirmed how nice it was that the foreigners were kind to her son.

For a man understood to be a simpleton, Arjun is remarkably effective at navigating the nuances of cross-cultural customer service. This alignment of circumstances would seem to present an obvious paradox, but critically his mother does not experience it as such. She loves her son, and she tells anyone who will listen how glad she is to have him back at home. Nevertheless—somehow—she perceives remarkably little about him. In the places that should be filled by meaning, she sees instead actions without purpose and efficacy without understanding. These assessments are conspicuous and difficult to explain. After all, Arjun's mother is a lodger of foreign tourists by trade, and she is surrounded constantly by people she does not understand. Most of her guests speak languages that she doesn't know, and they all have habits and dispositions that she finds strange. In a very real way, her livelihood is built from the gaps left by cultural and linguistic difference, and yet she does not hesitate to fill these gaps with meaning, or at least the possibility of it. On one occasion, she even pressed me with obvious amusement to explain why foreigners are so eager to carry heavy backpacks up a mountain and call it a "vacation." In the end, she concluded it must have something to do with "American culture." In this capacity and countless others, her ways of not knowing her guests are very different from her ways of not knowing her son.

On one particular visit, for example, I arrived to find Arjun's mother stumbling over herself to explain a complicated bill to a Japanese tourist. The conversation wasn't going well, and both of them were struggling to maintain their good humor. Her guest was upset, and it wasn't clear to her why. This led her to speculate urgently about the contents of his mind. The problem, she guessed, had something to do with how lodging for his porters had been tallied, but that's as far as she could get. In these moments of breakdown, the only thing she had at her disposal was a vast set of heuristics built through years of trial and error. She was adamant, for example, that one should never smile too much at Japanese people when they are feeling frustrated. "It makes them mad," she said. "That's all I know." In this regard, though her guest was profoundly foreign to her, his foreignness had in its own way come to be something familiar. It served not only to separate her from him but also to connect them together through a shared experience of mutual opacity: "I don't understand him, and he knows I don't understand him, and I know that he knows that I don't understand him . . . ," she explained with a laugh. About Arjun, her reflections are much simpler. "He's dumb, poor thing. He knows his desires, but he understands nothing else."

It is as if there is a single rule that defines for Arjun's family how everything he does should be interpreted: namely, his actions are only and exactly what they appear to be. They do not reveal something else about him, they do not indicate his state of mind, and they do not communicate his intentions or goals in anything but the most immediate sense. When Arjun gets on the roof to manipulate the solar panels, for example, his actions do not demonstrate that he understands electrical circuits; when he spends more than an hour each morning styling his hair and selecting his clothes, his choices do not reveal any interest in fashion; when he reads newspapers, journals, and magazines, his time spent does not suggest that he might be knowledgeable about politics and current events. Indeed, even as Arjun fills notebook after notebook with a staggering diversity of words and phrases, the fact that he can do so does not even demonstrate that he has access to language. Instead, when Arjun writes, his family perceives only and exactly that. He is not studying, he is not recording, and he is not communicating. He is merely applying ink to a sheet of paper, and nothing more.

Deaf people worldwide live amidst broad patterns of misrecognition, but these constraints on how Arjun's actions can be interpreted are especially perplexing. As I will argue in the coming pages, understanding them properly requires careful attention to the details of his life and context. Nepali ways of not-knowing the deaf are deeply regional in their organization, and any other cultural configuration—built on any other set of epistemological practices, any other social architecture of perception, or any other history of discourse— could have situated Arjun in completely different circumstances. Indeed, this possibility that things could have been very different for Arjun is exactly what Georges-Louis Leclerc, comte de Buffon, described in his *Natural History*. In this massively ambitious catalog of everything, Leclerc includes the story of a young man in eighteenth-century France who, after more than twenty years of life, comes to hear and speak for the first time. What shocks his family and community, however, is less his miraculous cure than the revelations that come after:

> A young man twenty-three to twenty-four years old, son of a craftsman of Chartres, deaf and dumb from birth, suddenly began to speak, to the great astonishment of all the city. It was known to him that some three or four months before he had heard the sound of bells, and had been extremely surprised by this new and unfamiliar sensation. Then a kind of water escaped his left ear, and he began to hear perfectly in both ears: for three or four months he listened without saying anything, and maturing in pronunciation and ideas of the words, and finally he thought himself able to break the silence, and it is said that he spoke though still imperfectly.
>
> Skilled theologians immediately questioned him about his past state, and unraveled their main issues about God, the soul, the moral goodness or evil actions. He did not seem to have pushed his thoughts far.
>
> Although born of literate Catholic parents, he attended Mass, and he was there instructed to make the sign of the cross and kneel in the capacity of a man who prays, he never had attached to all this any intention or other meaning; he knew not distinctly what it was that is death, and he never thought on it. (Buffon 1801, 231; see also Rée 1999, 92, for a different analysis thereof)

Though Leclerc's anonymous young deaf man kneeled, took communion, and moved his lips in prayer, he did not in fact believe; he had no thoughts of death or what came after and no remembrance of Christ's suffering. Instead, his religious devotion was mere replication. This minimal physicality was a sufficient mimesis because he found no reason to see the acts of those around him as anything more. There are clear echoes here of Arjun's life, though the players and assumptions are conspicuously reversed. Just as Arjun's parents never seem to question the constraints they perceive on the access Arjun has to everything that surrounds him, these parents of Chartres were horrified to learn that their son had copied their behaviors without also sharing their sense of purpose. Though these cases are built on diametrically opposed assessments of the deaf, they are unified by a single human tendency: people—when faced with the fact of actors and actions—maintain assumptions about the entailments of agency that are remarkably stable across time. Through a lifetime of interactions and potential disruptions, their intuitions perdure.

In my presence at least, the only person who ever expressed any doubt over these assessments of Arjun was Suddha, and her way of talking about her husband offers something of an exception to clarify the rule. Though her role as a young daughter-in-law in a busy household made it logistically difficult for me to interview her at any length, she was nevertheless always eager to talk. She stopped me repeatedly in passing moments, invariably to ask the same very pointed question: How could she know what Arjun is thinking? Initially, I found this a very strange question for her to be asking. Suddha is actually reasonably proficient as a signer. She is the only person in the immediate area who can communicate effectively with Arjun about anything more than basic topics. Nevertheless, this fact of access seems not to make her assessments any more straightforward. The hesitation she feels serves to color the intimacy the two of them share.

Arjun and Suddha often spend their evenings together in a gazebo adjoining the main house. Long after everyone else has gone to bed, they huddle close and talk for hours in the signed-language equivalent of hushed tones. To anyone listening, their interactions are silent, punctuated only by frequent laughter. To see them, however, is to realize how animated their time together is. On these nights, they occupy a space that is strikingly out of step with the rest of the hotel's aesthetic. It is wallpapered with bold and garish posters, each juxtaposing an oversaturated stock image with an incongruous bit of reappropriated text. One photo of Alpine cottages bears the subtitle "Silence is consent," for example, and another, featuring a basket of kittens, declares prominently that "The family is more sacred than the state." Arjun's favorite poster involves an assortment of traditionally dressed foreign natives lined up above the words "Love conquers all." Arjun's parents hate the gazebo and its loud colors. The fact that it even exists is a clear concession to his sense of style and a remembrance of his life in Kathmandu. For precisely this reason, perhaps, Arjun and Suddha prefer it to any other part of the hotel. When I asked each of them separately why they spent so much time there, both of them described it as the one place they could truly be alone. To outward appearances, at least, this is a very familiar scene: here is a young couple, fully enamored with each other, talking (as Arjun later explained to me) about their dreams for the future. When I asked Suddha about these long conversations, however, her response was heartfelt but also ambivalent and pained: "I like talking with him. We can talk all night. But, I don't know how much he understands. I think he does, a lot of it. But how can this be known?"

Evaluations of other minds are by necessity engagements with lacunae, the projection of content into gaps. When it comes to Arjun, however, very little is taken for granted to fill that space. He would seem to demonstrate the outward signs of a cognitively complex and socially engaged existence, and yet his family believes him to have no such access to their world. Even Suddha, who can understand Arjun perfectly well in the course of a normal conversation, is filled with anxiety by the ambiguity of what stands *behind* the things he says. How is it that all these people know so little about Arjun's mind? Or, rather, how is it that they know so much, so strangely? What motivates and maintains this claim of conspicuous absence that seems so plainly dissonant with Arjun's visible behaviors? And why is it that itinerant foreign backpackers, contextually dislocated and culturally illiterate, uniformly experience Arjun's intelligence so differently than does his kin?

At least as far as I could ever tell, there was never anything about Arjun more particular than his deafness that led his neighbors and family members to understand him in such consistently marginal terms. To the contrary, everyone I talked to seemed to agree that he is exceptionally capable . . . as far as deaf people go. This compliment and its caveat formed a very familiar two-part refrain in my conversations with the hearing. Deaf people, it would seem, are never *typical* for those who know them. They are always above average, at least within the space of expectation carved by their deafness. This way of talking about the deaf was a concession, I think, one meant to demonstrate generosity to the marginal without ever opening the question of whether the logic of marginality itself might be cruel and misattributed. When pressed, my sources would usually agree that as a matter of principle deaf people could be capable of anything, but they would do so reluctantly. Perhaps hospitals in foreign countries could somehow augment deaf capacities, they would say, but at least around here the long tail of possibility is occupied only by exceptions to the rule.

This question of exceptions haunts both deaf people and deaf political movements. Helen Keller, for example, is at least as famous in rural Nepal as she is in urban America. This is likely due to her designation in the government social studies textbooks as a "Great Person in History." Even decades after leaving school, hearing people would recite for me with great enthusiasm the one-sentence biography they had learned by rote: *Helen Keller was the first deaf and blind woman in the world to earn a bachelor's degree*. Though this prominence in the curriculum was undoubtedly meant as a gesture of inclusion towards people with disabilities, in practice it has become more a liability than an asset for deaf Nepal. Keller's life was indeed remarkable. She was centrally involved in many of the twentieth century's most important transformations in education, labor, and personhood. Without this context, however, her biography serves only to emphasize how singular she was as an educated individual. It is a beautiful and compelling story, but when familiar things like bachelor's degrees demand nothing less than international greatness from the deaf, it is far too easy to expect very little from the deaf boy or deaf girl living next door.

The cold reality is that these low expectations in fact often come to be self-fulfilling. Nepal is a country with very little public infrastructure, and its economic circumstances are especially stark for deaf children. Most never gain access to specialized education, and even those who do often have very little interaction with deaf adults. Consequently, only a small percentage of deaf people in Nepal ever learn Nepali Sign Language. Some come to speak and understand spoken Nepali through its visual cues—so-called "lipreading"—but acquiring language in this way is both arduous and technical. For most deaf Nepalis most of the time, the languages that surround them are met only as fragments and patches. As a result, the majority of Nepal's deaf children grow up never learning *any* language fluently. The cognitive and social effects of this isolation are devastating (Mayberry and Eichen 1991; Meier 1991; Dyssegaard 2000; Crowe, Gimire, and Trollo 2016).

Arjun, of course, is anything but linguistically isolated, but it is here that we might begin to see the terms in which his ostensible inabilities are anticipated. In an environment of far too familiar linguistic deprivation, it is telling that the conversations I witnessed about him so often began and ended with the observation that he lacks "voice" (āwaj). This statement was always met with knowing nods and sighs of pity. In South Asia, there are few things more closely identified with a person's capacity to think, act, and accomplish than speech (Kunreuther 2006). Voice offers both a metaphor and the basic mechanism of social action, and to be without voice is thus to occupy both the symbol and the substance of an especially forceful kind of social paralysis. Much like the English word *dumb*, the word most commonly used to refer to the deaf in colloquial

Nepali — *lāṭo²* — also serves as a more general epithet for the stubborn and the stupid. This overlap has wide and consistent implications. In everything from folk tales to modern sitcoms, the deaf are paradigmatic fools.

It is worth noting that the same rules seem not to apply to the blind, however. When hearing people shared with me their day-to-day experiences with disability, their stories were filled with blind savants and deaf village idiots, blind holy men and deaf wretches, or blind friends and deaf people who just happened to live nearby. The blind were frequently the heroes or villains of the tales I heard, while the deaf typically had too little presence of self to amount to either. Blindness was an affliction, to be sure, but in the accounts I heard, its basis of suffering was often tempered by something more fundamentally positive: a transcendence above material banalities, an access to a truer wisdom, or even a higher order of sense perception (cf. Miles 2001). A distant cousin of Arjun's, for example, is both blind and well known in the area as a skilled musician. The people I asked about him were vehement that he would be nowhere near as talented as he is if he could see. As Arjun's mother put it, "He can hear things that others can't." When I asked her if Arjun could likewise *see* things that she and I couldn't, she merely seemed confused. I asked again, and she thought for a moment before finally replying, "Like what?" Indeed, where blindness is most notable for its power to transform, deafness is perceived merely as a lack.

These narrative framings are powerful, but in the rest of this chapter I will argue that ideologies are never enough to explain how the hearing experience deafness. Instead, to know Arjun is to know him through a range of social entanglements. He is not only deaf but also a son, a husband, and a hotel owner, and his every encounter with those around him is shaped by the intersections of these relationships. Any claim about Arjun as a deaf man must likewise be read in the context of these diverse frameworks of coherence: as a tutor for deaf children, as a consumer of middle-class lifestyle goods, as an employer in the tourism service industry, as a young husband very much in love, and as a potential father ambivalent about the future. Amidst these patterned histories of interaction, it is not simply that Arjun's family members *think* he is a simpleton; they experience him as such at some moments but not at others, and they persist in maintaining this organization of their experiences throughout the course of

---

2.   As in many other places, the term most often translated as "the deaf" in Nepal more literally means "the mute," as it is their inability to speak rather than their inability to hear that serves to define the class.

a lifetime of interactions with him. Though this separation of identity and efficacy may seem paradoxical, it is ultimately a tension basic to the problem of personhood. The deafness of Arjun is not uniform but rather carves a shape in space and time.

Arjun's language notebooks offer a particularly clear illustration of how this complexity unfolds in context. Over months and years, these books have been filled with a vast collection of words and phrases shared by a diversity of native speakers, and as guides to foreign languages they have become a tremendous resource to the family business. Everyone in the household relies on them for the day-to-day demands of communicating with customers. At any given moment, a dozen different notebooks will lie scattered about the public spaces of the hotel, conspicuously disruptive of the otherwise tidy aesthetic. Given how disorganized the notebooks are, it is remarkable to me that anyone could ever find them useful, but Arjun knows the contents of each book intimately. Increasingly, his parents do too. They know, for example, that many words and phrases about food in Korean can be found at the end of the hardback with the eagle on the cover, and that the especially tattered blue notebook is mostly French. On one occasion, I even saw Arjun's mother frantically search the reception desk in a frustrated rage when she couldn't find the notebooks. She needed to explain a particularly complicated bill to a tourist, and she was lost without the translations they offered. These engagements demonstrate an unexpected separation between the efficacy of the things that Arjun *does* and the sort of person he is assumed to *be*. Arjun's notebooks *work*, and they are *useful* as guides to foreign languages, but nevertheless they do not render his interior complexity visible. Instead, not knowing Arjun is a complexly structured act, mediated by elaborate patterns of what the hearing do and don't see about him.

However relentless narratives about Arjun and his abilities might seem to be, the way his family members perceive him in social context does not ultimately depend on what he is and isn't able to *do*. To properly understand these dynamics, we need to think about Arjun and his opacity as an ethnographic problem. The issue here is far more layered and far more broadly involved than any survey of attitudes about deafness can reveal. Instead, Arjun is experienced by those around him through countless daily interactions, each individually minuscule and ideologically habituated. Though it is convenient to characterize these interactions in broad terms—pity, derision, misrecognition, dismissal, neglect—I think it is also a mistake. These descriptive organizations are coherent only retrospectively, and they serve more generally to erase the patterns of perception and notice that carve out a space for Arjun's deafness in the hearing world. In the course of any given day, Arjun moves through complexly organized regimes of coherence and incoherence, recognition and invisibility, and specificity and lack. It is these patterned ways of seeing, more than any single narrative, that shape how he is knowable to those around him.

LINGUISTIC DILEMMAS

To trace these patterns of perception from Arjun's perspective, we need look no further than the dilemma he faces in language. Arjun is one of the roughly five thousand fluent speakers of Nepali Sign Language (NSL). It is, in every respect, his primary language. It is the language he prefers for political debate, and it is the language he swears in when he drops something heavy on his foot. Nobody in Arjun's family has ever encountered NSL except through him, and only Suddha has come to understand it with any degree of competency. There is nothing odd about these limitations on their access. Like all languages, NSL is something that must be learned to be known. It is anchored to the very particular histories of a very particular speech community in Kathmandu, and using it effectively requires a specific and acquired knowledge of vocabulary, grammar, and discursive conventions. It is not, in other words, just pantomime.

What is strange is that no one in Arjun's family really seems to know that. They don't know, specifically, that Arjun knows a language that they do not. They can communicate with him effectively enough about basic topics in something that *feels* like signing to them, so the question of actually *learning* NSL doesn't really occur to them as necessary. Instead, their communication is built from what they call "natural signs": correspondences of visual form and meaning that strike them as obvious enough to be taken for granted. To reference a cow, for example, they simply think about what a cow looks like—it has horns—and they recreate these features visually in hopes of communicating the concept. Though some limited formal conventions have started to emerge within the household, the bulk of what Arjun's family members call "sign language" is assembled from precisely this kind of flexible creativity. The family "cow" might be referenced by one gestural shape one day and another the next, and all claims, questions, or commands about a particular cow in the here-and-now tend to be limited to visually oriented adjectives and a handful of very kinetic verbs. Arjun's family members would likely have no difficulty indicating that their particular cow has bolted off towards the south, for example, but they would struggle to explain that they regard cows generally as sacred because they embody the selfless giving of motherhood. According to this framework of expectations, signing functions much like a game of charades, and the set of visual intuitions that make this game possible comprise the entire scope of what Arjun's family members understand his language to be.

Suddha offers a limited exception to this very ad hoc way of engaging the question of NSL, but even her signing slides surprisingly easily between aspects of the Kathmandu standard she has picked up from Arjun and her own real-time innovations. More importantly even, she makes no distinction whatsoever between these two very different circumscriptions of Arjun's linguistic experiences. Indeed, when I asked Suddha why she thought she was able to communicate with her husband better than anyone else could, she made no mention of having *learned* his language or anything else. Instead, she noted that she and Arjun were close, and she speculated that this closeness caused their talk to "fit" (*najik bhaera hāmro kurā milchha*). Contrary to a broader intuition in Nepal that language maps ethnic identity (see chapter 3), Arjun's signing is experienced even by those closest to him as something that needs neither history nor community to work. That's the point. As with everything else about him, Arjun's communicative practices are perceived as broadly self-evident, emergent unmediated from his present experiential state and thus free of anything resembling the self-consciousness necessary for explicit convention. When Arjun's family members call his signs "natural," then, what they are saying is that they demonstrate neither more nor less than the universal human capacity to find meaning in the visual contours of the world.

The most remarkable fact is that this understanding *does* work for them, sort of. It works because of a very particular fact about sign language signs: in context, signs often *resemble* the things they mean. They are not freely gestural, but they are frequently *iconic*. The NSL dictionary entries for "elephant," "water," "mountain," "red," and "trekking porter," for example, bear striking similarities to qualities of these things that are salient to deaf and hearing Nepalis alike (figures 1–5).[3] Elephants have trunks, water is poured into the mouth, mountains make a triangular shape, red powder is frequently placed between the eyes,

---

3. All line drawings of NSL signs in this book were created by Pratigya Shakya for the *Nepali Sign Language Dictionary* (Nepali Sign Language National Development Committee 2003), discussed in greater detail in chapter 3.

and porters carry loads with a strap across their foreheads. Fast and fluent signing is always opaque to outsiders, but in isolation many well-formed sentences aren't. This is especially true when they are assembled carefully in ways meant to be accessible to the hearing. To precisely these ends, when Arjun signs with his family, he must always be cognizant of how they interpret his signs, and he uses these judgments to select vocabulary that he expects will make him easily

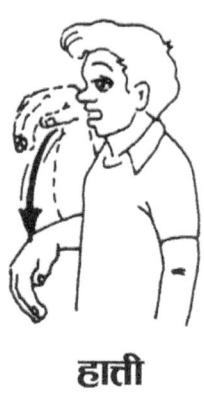
हात्ती

Figure 1. ELEPHANT

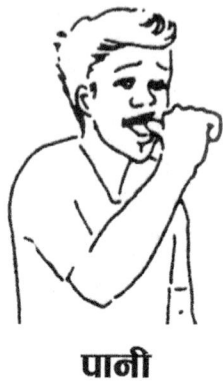
पानी

Figure 2. WATER

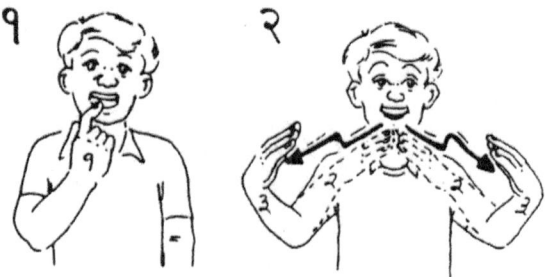

हिमाल

Figure 3. MOUNTAIN

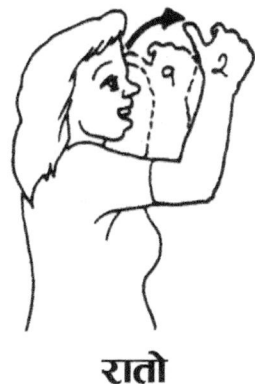

राेतो

Figure 4. RED

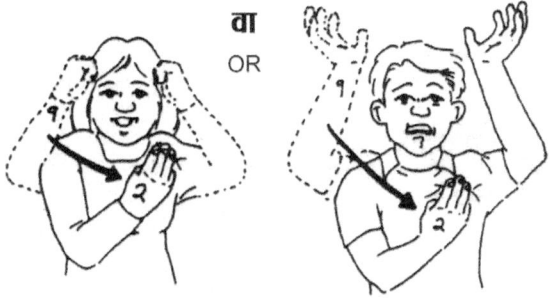

भरीया/कुल्ली

Figure 5. PORTER

understood. In these moments, I don't think it is useful or interesting to suggest that these family members are speaking a "language," least of all NSL; but what about Arjun? How should we think about *his* communicative practices as they engage his nondeaf family? Arjun's language at home is clearly different to his language in Kathmandu, but it is much more difficult to say exactly how.

Deaf languages have existed as far back as our records go, but it was not until the 1960s that hearing people really started to *notice* them consistently. People knew, of course, that the deaf sometimes used their hands to communicate, and philosophers as far back as Plato even used this fact to illustrate far-reaching claims about the nature of the human mind (Plato 2008). Yet, even as scholars saw deaf people *using* sign, they paid remarkably little attention to the fact of sign itself. Instead, across this long history, signing was taken for granted as something inevitable, not built from anything contextual or historically particular but rather a universal set of natural gestures available to anyone with eyes. There was nothing, in other words, particularly deaf about sign, except perhaps for the fact that deaf people needed it. Now, in linguistically minded circles at least, it is widely understood that signed languages are indeed languages in every technical and functional sense. They have grammars, vocabularies, and histories of change that are uniquely their own. All of these things were always there, of course. They might have been noticed at any time, but it wasn't until the hearing started looking for deaf language that it came to be seen.

As a consequence of this history, perhaps, the name "Nepali Sign Language" has led many to assume that NSL draws its base from spoken Nepali, translating an otherwise acoustic language into a manual and visual medium. This is flatly incorrect. In reality, NSL seems to have emerged directly from its earliest community of deaf users, with no clear hereditary links to any other language, spoken or signed. That's not to say that speakers of NSL lack access to the other languages around them. To the contrary, they are surrounded constantly by Nepali and other spoken languages, and, as a direct consequence of this environment, their language possesses numerous conventions for drawing spoken-language words into the signing channel. Fingerspelling, for example, allows signers to recreate letter sequences from either the Roman or the Devanagari alphabets manually, but its use is limited largely to loan words and proper nouns. A signer might fingerspell the name P-E-T-E-R to introduce me, for example, but any further account of my being hearing, American, an anthropologist, and so on, would use signs with no ties to the structure of either Nepali or English. Apart from these very limited interfaces designed explicitly to shift words across modalities, the two languages share effectively zero formal structure. Instead, NSL's linguistic history is built from distinctly deaf histories of interaction.

In Darjeeling, a Nepali-speaking city in India, for example, deaf signers do not use NSL but instead *another* language that is itself also largely autonomous (R. J. Johnson and Johnson 2016). Owing to the rise in recent years of deaf YouTube channels, however, Kathmandu- and Darjeeling-based signers are often able to communicate with each other in a pidgin drawn from American Sign Language (ASL). American Sign Language and British Sign Language, meanwhile, bear little resemblance to each other, despite their shared context of English. Instead, ASL is closely related to the languages used by signers in both France and Russia, and as a consequence of this history deaf Nepalis might have an easier time communicating with deaf Russians than with their neighbors across the Indian border to the south or the Chinese border to the north. The geography here gets complicated very quickly, but there is no explanation for its shape more general than history. The distribution of linguistic diversity around the world is the consequence of accumulated patterns of migration and exchange, and sometimes these patterns are very different for the deaf than for the hearing. It is these complex social relationships, ultimately, that Arjun's family members fail to see, and it is the absence of this social history that allows his language to appear as no more than gesture.

In this regard, Arjun's family members are not alone. Since the rise of signed language linguistics in the 1960s and 1970s, a great deal of ink has been spilled trying to disambiguate language from gesture. Since Arjun's family members have never learned NSL as a language, what they use to communicate with him would generally be understood as gestural, though perhaps also partially conventionalized enough to constitute what has been called a "homesign system" (Senghas and Coppola 2001; Goldin-Meadow 2005b; Brentari et al. 2012). The idea here would be that Arjun participates in two distinct though sometimes blended communicative systems. The first would be a constraint-driven architecture of arbitrary rules and forms, comprising grammar and vocabulary in the traditional sense. The second, in contrast, would be an emergent system of pantomime, which imagines communication much more broadly as a series of creatively functional techniques rather than linguistic code. To this bifurcated analysis, NSL is exactly the first system disambiguated from the second. NSL is, specifically, the thing fluent signers do with each other and not what happens at the boundaries of deaf and hearing worlds. What extent of transparency exists in NSL proper then would be a relic of its gestural past, a historical legacy of etymological processes that has been supplanted by and shouldn't be confused with the real stuff of linguistic structure. In this analysis, sign language is language precisely to the extent that it has ceased to be gestural.

The trouble is, it is not at all clear that this distinction between language and gesture is meaningfully present in what Arjun does when he signs. Consider the sign for "water" (figure 2 above). Is it a sign or a gesture? It is used identically by both Arjun and his family members, and thus it is impossible to make a distinction in purely formal terms. Yet, clearly, there is a great deal at stake in being able to say that Arjun knows NSL but his family members do not. We could argue, perhaps, that the formational properties of WATER constitute a linguistic lexical item for Arjun but a pantomimed gesture for his family members (or, perhaps, a lexical item in Kathmandu but a gesture at home), but at the end of it all, it is not obvious what these asymmetries of function accomplish for us analytically. This demands a complex analysis, but it also boils down to a simple fact: though the theoretical stakes of making these two speech contexts categorically different are very high, I can't say that I ever saw Arjun sign something to his parents that wouldn't have been a well-formed sentence in Kathmandu as well. NSL is governed by a rich and multiply layered body of conventions, but it is remarkably difficult to outline the boundaries around it.

This ambiguity puts Arjun in a difficult position. Because his family members can understand what he is saying some of the time, seemingly without effort or foreknowledge, the moments in which they don't take on a strange perceptual salience. As an experience of the senses, the partial access Arjun's family members have to NSL stands in sharp contrast to the total opacity of Japanese, English, or French. This difference between spoken and signed language was often explicit in my interviews with the hearing. Arjun and I, as proficient signers, generally spoke to each other in a standard dialect of Kathmandu NSL, full of lexical, syntactic, and discursive conventions that are unknown by and thus inaccessible to Arjun's mother. Yet, on more than one occasion, she commented that the reason she could not understand us was because we were signing "too fast." When slowing down the conversation didn't help, she suggested that perhaps our time in Kathmandu had made our thinking sloppy. The words and signs that she cannot extract from Arjun's speech become noise in a signal otherwise assumed to be transparent. Arjun's language, in this sense, is both too familiar and too alien to be identified as an independent linguistic form like Nepali, English, Japanese, or Gurung. Instead, it appears as a prosthesis—a way for the deaf to access not *language* but rather the *effects* of language in the hearing world. The idea that Arjun's signing could be conventional or even grammatical simply doesn't feel necessary to his family to explain the fact that it *works*.

This places both Arjun's family members and the linguists of signed languages in precisely the same epistemological dilemma: attempts to disambiguate signed language from signed gestures must necessarily turn to questions of history, of why a sign and a meaning serve to correspond. The NSL sign for "water" and the idiosyncratic gesture occasionally used by Arjun's family are visually identical, even as they emerge from very different histories of use. They cannot be distinguished from each other as forms unto themselves but rather only through attention to the processes by which each came to be. Because signed language and signed gesture coexist so seamlessly in linguistic practice, however, Arjun's family members are at risk of perceiving the particularity of neither. Ultimately, they take their lack of comprehension to indicate a lack of content. They don't know that they don't know sign language.

We can now see Arjun's dilemma in its sharpest light: to be effective as a signer with his family, he must organize his speech in a way that narrows the conventional dimensions of his language radically. He must bear the burden of transparency for everyone around him, anchoring his words and expressions exclusively to a here-and-now of shared perception and memory. He must circumscribe his language to a history no larger than the one occupied by those immediately present. He must deny everything that makes NSL particular to a time, place, and community of practice. He must, in other words, confirm for his family members exactly what they already believe: that sign language is a transparent organization of basic shared experiences. This is profoundly unsatisfying for Arjun, to be sure. Nevertheless, it is a bind characteristic of being deaf in hearing worlds.

MAKING *SENSE*

As an interface between deaf and hearing worlds, Arjun's language is least well known when it is most easily understood. These paradoxical circumstances are organized by the very unusual conditions of interpretability that attend to NSL signs in context. Arjun may, at his discretion, present his language to those around him in ways that make it remarkably easy for nonsigners to understand, but in so doing he erases everything that is most particular about himself. This self-effacement is something that frustrates him, but being understood is often simply the more pressing necessity. By the weight of these accumulated moments, however, Arjun's family members settle into habituated patterns of seeing, anchored by their experiences of him as someone inevitably transparent. In the course of this perceptual history, their assessments of his abilities need not be hoisted on the back of particular narratives about disability because they feel already real enough to be taken for granted simply by the alignment of circumstances.

Here, we begin to see the shape of a much more general ethnographic theme. Though discursive framings are of course important to Arjun's broader story, they fail ultimately to explain his very unusual place in his family. Deafness is not an *idea* underwriting cultural patterns of behavior. Instead, Arjun's experiences as a deaf man take their shape from the interactions of what those around him do and don't perceive in the spaces that they cannot directly see. In this regard, what constitutes Arjun as an unusual figure in hearing contexts is not the set of beliefs about him but rather the elaborate and particular dynamic of perception that makes him known. To track this cultural dynamic effectively, we need a better way of understanding the entanglements that establish people like Arjun and Suddha, things like dictionaries and solar panels, and unifying abstractions like language, intention, and meaning in relation to one another. We need to know, in other words, how it is that Arjun and his deafness take shape as objects of experience in hearing places.

Arjun's notebooks are an especially clear demonstration of this problem, highlighting the capacity of things to sometimes absorb and sometimes reflect the traces of their own social histories. From this starting point, we can begin to trace the terms by which the paradox of Arjun's identity and public efficacy is maintained. No one denies that Arjun's notebooks are useful, but this fact of utility does not force the hearing people in his life to evaluate the conditions of their useful possibility. Instead, they are experienced in terms shaped by the perception of a more fundamental lack within them. "They are only empty words," his mother once told me. "He has a good eye, and a good hand, and he can make [the letters] beautifully. But there isn't any *sense* in them." In this explanation, the word "sense" is especially conspicuous; it is not a gloss of a Nepali term but rather a loan from English, one that has taken on very distinct connotations in the contexts in which I encountered it. A person might be said to lack *sense* if he or she does foolish things, but equally the word might be applied to someone in a coma. In this alignment, what *sense* describes is something somewhere at the intersections of the sens*ible* and the sens*ing*.

Popular Hindi movies, for example, are often said to be high on production value, violence, and sex, but very low on *sense*. When I asked a friend (as many surely have before me) why a gangster started dancing in the middle of an epic gun battle, he responded dismissively: "Because the woman started dancing. There's no *sense* beyond that." He was directing my attention, in other words, to a kind of unity that exists from frame to frame but that is absent from scene to scene. In service of this distinction, *sense* reveals to us how actions are motivated and how events are tied to broader histories of meaning, offering a second-order coherence to the world shaped by perception and its first-order experience of things. More specifically, what *sense* articulates is a recognition that things acquire the basis of their coherence from contexts larger than themselves. The word *sense* was frequently invoked by the hearing people I interviewed in this new and reorganized meaning. They used it to explain not only the deaf people in their lives, but also deaf actions, deaf effects, and the things the deaf have made. In this diversity of manifestations, what *sense* reveals is the engagements inherent among people and things, and thus its absence for the deaf implies not randomness but rather a lack of sensitivity to higher orders of context.

Consequently, when Arjun's mother describes her son as someone who lacks "sense," what she is saying is that she perceives something in him to be *missing*. She perceives, in other words, an absence where a presence should be. Though it is hard to identify exactly what form this presence ought to take, there is no question, I think, that it incorporates some aspect of his interiority. At its simplest, what Arjun lacks for those around him is the thing that would cause them to speculate about how to link his internal states to his observable behaviors. For example, if Arjun had *sense*, his family members would see purpose, knowledge, and agency in his tendency to fiddle with the solar panels. Instead, all they see is fiddling. This is a very unusual conditioning of perception. The difference between a wink and a twitch may be impossible to articulate concretely, but the capacity to perceive this difference in context is nevertheless precisely what makes social phenomena possible. It is a felt presence inhabiting actions, intangible but critical to how we engage the social world. This term "presence" has a long and tangled history in research on the nature of consciousness, but I am adopting it here for more basic and more overtly ethnographic ends: in social context, intentions are things; drives are real; the abstractions that people attribute to the world are just as consequential as any material form. The contours by which these shared objects of experience go seen or unseen ultimately determine how we identify what is most profoundly human in others. *Sense*, in this regard, is a very particular kind of substantiating presence, felt as real within the objects of hearing perception. About Arjun, for reasons that we must make clear, no such presence is perceived to exist.

It is this same encounter with emptiness that haunts Arjun's notebooks, and to understand the broader question of his senselessness we must understand the very contextual terms in which these notebooks are experienced. As tools for accessing foreign languages, Arjun's notebooks are convenient, accurate, and useful. As the product of a deaf individual, however, they take on characteristics that go beyond questions of mere utility. To Arjun's mother, for example, the fact that her son's notebooks *work* does not disrupt her intuition that they are filled

with what she calls "*nakalī* [counterfeit/duplicate] letters." The phrasing here
is evocative, undoubtedly meant to carry with it imagery of the fake currency
notes and knock-off electronics that infuse the region from across the nearby
Chinese border. Though counterfeit things may be indistinguishable from the
originals that they imitate, they are ultimately not *real* in some fundamental
way, and this lack of realness stands as a tangible risk to anyone who mistakes
them as such. The same word is used to describe inauthentic documents that are
rejected by bureaucracies, for example, or to warn men against overly "fashionable" women (Shneiderman 2014). Critically, what distinguishes the real from
the *nakalī* is not any particular material property but rather a hidden but inescapably consequential social history, experienced as a basic and tangible part
of things as they occupy the world. In these same terms, what is missing from
Arjun's notebooks is not attributable to any dimension of form or function.
Rather, Arjun's notebooks are *nakalī* because they were made by Arjun.

What this framing of Arjun's notebooks reflects is a way of relating to the
ambiguities inherent in the experience of others. This question of the *nakalī* is
rooted in contemporary Nepal by histories that expand far beyond deafness.
Everywhere, people are concerned that things are not as they seem. The anxiety is tangible, reflected in murmurs of conspiracy and unexpected spasms of
public violence. These are hard times, and—as it was constantly articulated to
me—even the most mundane decisions are made dangerous by a steady tension
between real things and fake things and the increasing difficulties inherent in
distinguishing the two. To a properly attentive mind, everything should be an
object of scrutiny, from fake cookware that might explode and kill families to
fake job advertisements that leave migrant workers stranded without documentation in hostile foreign countries. In these everyday moments, knowing how to
tell if something presented as real is *actually* real can be mortally urgent.

Primetime sitcoms like *Jire Khursānī* (Hot Pepper) and *Tito Satya* (Bitter
Truth) have leveraged this social dilemma into a distinct genre of satire, which
articulates socioeconomic development as a conquest of the naïve by the savvy.
Modernity, in this expression, is about knowing how to distinguish the actual
from the simulated and, moreover, about the public ridicule that comes from
failing to make these distinctions appropriately. The fate of those who lack
such knowledge was demonstrated particularly clearly in one episode of *Tito
Satya* that aired shortly after the end of Nepal's decade-long civil war. The story
centered on a middle-aged couple visiting Kathmandu for the first time from
some unnamed hinterland village. Dressed in traditional clothing and sporting

lowbrow nasal accents, the couple decided to go see a movie. They were, however, unaware that the film was fiction. At the story's climax, they were devastated to see their favorite actress perish in a fire, a horror borne by the conviction that they had just seen a woman *actually* burn to death. Compounding this trauma was the lackadaisical response of the other movie-goers, who chatted, threw popcorn, and jeered at the screen. When it became clear that no one else would speak out against this act of murder, the couple fled the theater in a panic. They threw themselves at the feet of a mannequin in a shop window and begged it to help them find a police officer to whom they might report the crime they had witnessed. When the mannequin didn't respond, the husband began to shake it furiously until it fell over and broke into pieces. Again horrified, they ran pell-mell down the street only to stumble upon—*deus ex machina*—their beloved and very alive actress strolling casually down the street. Overcome with both relief and confusion, they embraced her and told her what they had seen. She laughed, consoled them with maternal words, and explained that the film was only imaginary. The program's final shot returned to the couple, slumped with fatigue and trying hard to seem relieved. At this point, the credits began to roll, and cheerful music removed all doubts that this was indeed a happy ending.

Though *Tito Satya* is decidedly populist in its aesthetics, its plot-lines are frequently drawn (and transformed) from the highbrow echelons of world literature. This particular story bears striking resemblance to a segment in Gabriel García Márquez's *One Hundred Years of Solitude*, a novel popular among the class of young Nepali professionals who write teleplays. García Márquez tells a similar tale about a community of overly innocent villagers, faced with feelings of loss at the death of actors during a time of rapid modernization. In the Spanish-language novel, the story proceeds:

> Dazzled by so many and such marvelous inventions, the people of Macondo did not know where their amazement began. They stayed up all night looking at the pale electric bulbs fed by the plant that Aureliano Triste had brought back when the train made its second trip, and it took time and effort for them to grow accustomed to its obsessive toom-toom. They became indignant over the living images that the prosperous merchant Bruno Crespi projected in the theater with the lion-head ticket windows, for the character who had died and was buried in one film and for whose misfortune tears of affliction had been shed would reappear alive and transformed into an Arab in the next one. The audience, who paid two cents apiece to share the difficulties of the actors, would not tolerate that

outlandish fraud and they broke up the seats. The mayor, at the urging of Bruno
Crespi, explained in a proclamation that the cinema was a machine of illusions
that did not merit the emotional outbursts of the audience. With that discour-
aging explanation many felt that they had been the victims of some new and
showy gypsy business and they decided not to return to the movies, considering
that they already had too many troubles of their own to weep over the acted-out
misfortunes of imaginary beings. (García Márquez [1967] 2003, 223)

This misrecognition of imaginary beings as real ones is a familiar trope worldwide, but its effects in Macondo and Kathmandu are tellingly different. If this
is indeed a remix (cf. Greene 2001; Williams 2012), it is one that shows just
how little nostalgia contemporary Nepali scriptwriters have for the stakes of
innocence. In Macondo, the idea that sin and death should be forgiven so easily causes offense to the villagers, but critically it inspires them to a *collective*
rebellion. The lies of the silver screen are distressing, but ultimately they serve to
reaffirm the values of the community, rejecting those of outsiders and reiterat-
ing the autonomy of the local. For the Nepali couple, however, the experience
of mistaking the fake for the real is deeply isolating. This is a dark episode in
their lives, reminding them of the unbridgeable distance between the naïve and
the savvy. Though Macondo's villagers also fail to distinguish the real from the
fake, their credulity is depicted as a source of nobility and strength. In Nepal, the
same failures bring only dehumanizing trauma.

Nepali sitcoms of this genre have risen in prominence over the past two
decades along with a rising cynicism about the reliability of knowledge. There is
a self-consciousness about this shift, and people are quick to identify it if asked:
"*ājkal, bishwās chhaina*," they will say: these days, there is no belief/trust. The
absence of trust is familiar in the literatures on modernity: for many, the dis-
placements, shifts, and reorientations attendant on the spread of global capital
networks are experienced as an equal and anxious skepticism about both old and
new. In Nepal, this is revealed by a world of *Māobādīs* and *Khāobādīs*, Maoist
insurgents who are sometimes hard to distinguish from the imitators ("*khāo*" =
to eat) who use their name to commit grave acts of violence without a broader
political agenda. Concern about this kind of sourceless violence is widespread
and growing. In the wake of a particularly unprecedented spasm that left Kathmandu's most important mosque attacked and partially burned, for example,
even some of the rioters themselves insisted to me that the violence must have
been a ruse of the new king.

Critically, these anxieties have implications for finding good booze. As Frank Zappa almost said, to be a proper ethnic group in Nepal, one must not only make beer but also face accusations that one's beer is poisonous, prepared with unwholesome ingredients or sinister methods. The Tamang, it is alleged, make their *chhāṅg* with ground-up rubber sandals, and Newars make their *aylā* with shoe polish. Limbu women, we are told, make *toṅgbā* exclusively while menstruating, and Tibetans will sometimes ferment human bone. In their quest for locally made alcohol, many middle-aged men I knew spent tremendous effort to maintain complex networks of trust along these distinctly ethnic lines.[4] These anxieties emerge from the opacities of modern markets, and what is frustrating these days for many is that the old kinds of social networks increasingly fail to reveal what is and isn't as it seems (cf. Nakassis 2013). There's no use relying on taste or smell, either. As everyone savvy knows, acts of primary perception are just too fallible to be trusted; real alcohol is materially indistinguishable from the fake poisonous stuff.

Likewise, to separate the real from the fake in contemporary Kathmandu, it is not enough to know things through their observable properties. Rather, one must follow the substance to its source, walking through the transactions and translations that have brought the world's many things to be where they are. According to this frame of intuitions, the presence of an object is felt not just as a set of observable properties but, moreover, as an engagement with and consolidation of history. This basis of objecthood demands a very different kind of knowledge, one that displaces things from their ostensibly self-evident presence of form and reinvests them into variously large and variously conceptualized entanglements of context. Things are not self-sufficient unto themselves but rather exist as histories made tangible. When these histories are opaque, the *sense* of things is difficult to engage effectively.

As a way of framing the experience of social history in these terms, what *sense* reveals is thus an ontological intuition, one that extends the most perceptually tangible dimensions of forms, facts, and events into conceptual worlds. Without *sense*, things and actions are "empty," and this ever-present possibility of emptiness is what explains the gap between Arjun's obvious functional competencies and his ostensible deficits. When I asked Arjun's mother to elaborate

---

4.   Paul Manning (2012) notes similar elaborations over beer brands in Georgia, suggesting that alcohol might be particularly available as a materialization of opaque histories.

on what she meant when she called him *senseless*, for example, she illustrated with an example: "When he was very small, he would become angry and violent. He had no reason for it. It was just anger without a source." This was a period shortly before Arjun was sent to boarding school in Kathmandu. He was only five or six years old, but he would sometimes fight with the other children in the village, reportedly without cause. In the course of these fights, he would apparently become so enraged that his parents would lock him in his bedroom until he calmed down, sometimes hours later. It was this behavioral issue, more than any particular pedagogical instinct, that persuaded Arjun's parents to seek options away from home. "He was angry, sad, or happy without reason," his mother said. "The teachers at the school [in Kathmandu] have experience with this." Arjun has a very different memory of things, of course, though he was usually reluctant to talk about his childhood with me. He described being cruelly mocked by the other children in the neighborhood, and he recalled bitterly that his mother failed to do anything about it. Far from unmotivated, Arjun explains his behavior as driven by intense isolation, confusion, and fear. Nevertheless, because his private experience remains for his family members so inaccessible as an underlying organization of purpose, his actions appear without *sense*. As his mother put it, "He has a body but no intellect (*buddhi*)."[5]

Arjun's mother went on to describe another example meant to illustrate his lack of *sense*:

> The horses love Arjun, because they know he has no *sense*. When he is kind to them, it is only kindness. But when I am kind to the horses, they are suspicious. If I give them carrots or brush them, they know that it is because I will soon stick them with a syringe or make them carry a particularly fat tourist. But Arjun is simple (*sojho*). What he does is what he means (*usle je gareko, te matlab*).

This turn of phrase, stipulating an inherent equivalence between deaf actions and meanings, was ubiquitous in my interviews with the hearing. The intuition

---

5.   In Sanskrit philosophy, *buddhi* is generally presented in contrast to *manas*. In broad terms, both words mean "mind", but *manas* refers specifically to a lower-order responsiveness engaged by the material world. It is responsible for such things as ego-construction and attraction to objects. *Buddhi*, in contrast, describes a higher, inherently reflexive aspect of the mind that is attuned to an ultimate reality. A being with *manas* but no *buddhi* would be a zombie of sorts, potentially able to act coherently but without any sense of higher purpose.

that stands behind it serves to dampen any impulse within Arjun's family to fill in the gaps left by his outward behavior. It explains why even his most complexly instrumental actions nevertheless remain "empty" (*khāli*), as his family members so often said. There is simply no drive for them to populate the open spaces of their fragmentary experience where he is concerned with higher-order coherences. Arjun—as a person without *sense*—is only and exactly as he appears to be.

For the horses, *sense* is a capacity for guile, the possibility that a caregiver's inward state and outward expression might be intentionally mismatched for his or her own strategic ends. For personal experience, *sense* is appropriateness, the contextual link that explains affect as a manifestation of broader dynamics of emotion. For written language, *sense* is purpose, the use of text to constitute an act of communication that goes beyond the mere reproduction of form. Together, what these distinctions reveal is a sophisticated intuition made tangible in very everyday cultural practices. People in Nepal know that things never stand for themselves; they know there's always a greater story. *Sense* is the underlying intuition of this entanglement.[6] Though a copier and a writer may produce identical written forms on an identical page, only the writer has *sense* because only the writer has invested those forms with *intention*. In these terms, *sense* is the presence of agency congealed by social objects in context, a hidden logic that cannot be seen directly but nevertheless must be experienced as real for social actions and social things to cohere amidst the noise of perceptual realities. To participate in regimes of *sense* is thus to engage in a form of embodiment-for-others, presenting the self as sensitive to both the material and the social organizations of being simultaneously. This is, one might argue, a particularly sharp definition of culture, but critically it is one to which Arjun stands as an exception. Arjun does not have *sense* like others do because, as his family understands him, he does not allow for questions of existence to be mediated by social facts, histories, and regimes of shared perception. He is, instead, so radically transparent that preconceptions are unnecessary to know him.

---

6. *Sense* is, in this, notably related to Frege's use of the term (or, more accurately, the use of the term by Frege's translators) (Frege 1997). In the categories of South Asian philosophy, this is also (and perhaps more robustly) related to Bhartrihari's notion of *sphoṭa*, an expression of irreducible meaningful efficacy that emerges from language but cannot be reduced to the sum of its constituents (Rath 2000). In this distinctly South Asian vernacular, *sense*—like *sphoṭa*—is the whole that displaces its own parts (Coward 1997).

It is here that Arjun finds himself with respect to his family, exempt from all normal cultural assumptions that project actions into intentions, events into narratives, presences into things, and instances into categories. As a senseless self, Arjun is immediate, reactive, and imitative. He produces correctly things like kindness to animals, expressions of anger, and foreign words, but to those around him these actions neither require nor allow contextualization beyond an immediate frame of reference. Arjun treats the horses kindly, but his kindness is a disposition without purpose; he is angry, but his anger is affect without emotion; he writes, but his writing is code without content. Because Arjun's *behaviors* are experienced as so directly transparent, because they *feel* self-explanatory to those around him, there is no benefit to be had in speculating about higher-order coherences like purpose, meaning, or mind because—simply put—everything he does can be explained well enough without them. No matter what he does, his actions do not serve as *indications* of an extended self but rather stand, sufficient, as total facts. Arjun thus inhabits an unenviable place in a world of pure presences, one that denies consequence to everything except that which is immediately seen. He is an exception, in other words, to the general *sense* of things. In the most perverse and dehumanizing way possible, Arjun is completely free.

THE PRESENCE OF ARJUN

There is a piece to this story that still puzzles me. Arjun, for reasons I am only beginning to understand, shows no interest whatsoever in disabusing his family members of their misconceptions. This is unusual, to say the least. Over the last two decades especially, young and educated deaf people like Arjun have risen up as a collective movement, fighting to tear down the various attitudes, terminologies, and policies that push deaf voices into the margins. Under the banner of this new and boundlessly optimistic activism, the task of "awareness raising" (NSL: *thumb and index finger join at the temple, then separate as eyes open wide*) is consistently articulated as an almost sacred duty. Within these circles, stories about deaf people who are first identified as simpletons only to later shatter that characterization through some display of virtuosity have come to constitute something of a narrative genre in their own right. Arjun himself shared many such stories with me from his time in Kathmandu, and yet here at home—among the people most immediately consequential to his life—he was unexpectedly quiet. When I asked him why, he shrugged my questions off. When I asked if he wanted me to take any messages back to his friends in Kathmandu, he requested that I not tell anyone that I saw him. If I decided to write about him, he wanted me to change his name (which I have done).

Arjun is angry, particularly with his mother. The precise contours of this experience are likely too personal to be accessible to ethnography directly, except perhaps through Sapir's famous admonition that anthropologists need psychoanalysts (Sapir [1938] 2001). Whatever dynamics of mind and emotion might be at play, however, the particular ways in which the relationship between Arjun and his mother has broken down are telling: Arjun has elected to remain unintelligible. He has allowed his mother to persist in her nonperception of his mind, and in doing so he has excluded her from one of the most important identities in deaf organizations of kinship: the mother whose child has taught her what it really means to be deaf. In denying his mother access to that experience, he is keeping his world to himself.

Arjun's mother loves her son deeply. She talks about him constantly, and she worries about whether he is happy. And Arjun loves her too. He worries about her health, and in our conversations he wondered with unconcealed heartache about whether he will be able to care for her as she gets older. Though they frequently fight, he never once uttered a harsh word about her to me. His decision to leave her and everyone else in the dark about who he is thus cannot be dismissed as mere lack of care or interest. Instead, what we should see in this choice, and what we see consistently in Arjun's way of engaging with his family members, is something much more particularly deaf.

When I first met Arjun, he was preoccupied by an ambitious project to restructure his phrasebooks. As he explained to me, the purpose of this work was to replace the disorder that had accumulated over the previous few years with something more interesting and more useful. In their old form, Arjun's notebooks were organized by the chronology of their construction. When he met a new speaker of a foreign language willing to sit down with him for a few minutes, he would draw a horizontal line below where his previous work had ended, and he would proceed to elicit whatever words and phrases he could. Leafing through these old notebooks sequentially thus reveals a telling biography, cataloging the people Arjun met and the various vocabularies he happened to find interesting at the time. The new system, in contrast, would be organized by principles of meaning, each page designating a phrase or small group of words that could be populated with their particular instantiations in all the various languages he could encounter. He had started to implement this new system in his notebooks. Under a section header labeled "Smoking, drinking, and food," for example, one page contained the phrase "How much is a pack of cigarettes?" in eleven languages. Another page in another section asked "Where is the hospital?" in eight, and still another informed "Yaks do not live at this elevation" in English, Dutch, and Chinese. This new organization manifests a very different dimension of language as a social fact. In the old system, language is a contextual production issued by particular speakers at particular moments of history; in the new system, language is an almost mechanical alignment of forms and meanings.

So what do we make of this? Is Arjun's work to reorganize his language notebooks just an attempt to maximize their utility? Perhaps, but given the countless hours that he has poured into this project, it seems unlikely that the depth and unusual character of his focus are merely incidental. Is there, perhaps, something far more *deaf* about this engagement with language? I think so, but to see it I think we need an explicitly ethnographic analysis of Arjun's sensitivities to hearing patterns of perception.

In their new organization, Arjun's notebooks demonstrate a clear interest in the experience of specificity and difference. They carefully document the fact that Japanese, French, Dutch, and Australian speakers say the same things with different words. These various nationalities might all equivalently want a cup of tea or directions to the next town, for example, but they will express these meanings through different sequences of sound. Equivalent desires, in other words, often manifest as different kinds of linguistic behavior in context. To someone in the possession of a universal phrasebook, however, linguistic patterns of variation whittle down to something far more atomic and isolable. A German might ask to go to the hospital in a distinctly German way (and perhaps even for distinctly German reasons), but once stripped of these cultural and linguistic conventions such a request is potentially no more German than Korean, Hebrew, or Italian. Arjun's meticulous organization of these inscriptions is thus an act of systematic reduction, the making transparent of correspondence between forms and meanings that can, in the course of habitualized use, collapse into each other. Someone who wants to go to the hospital certainly has a story to tell, but the bare act of telling a story makes *sense* only through these lateral entanglements of social context. By reducing these phrases to their most bare equivalences, Arjun is making salient a very particular way of experiencing linguistic opacity. He is suggesting that, with the right frame of attention, acts of speech can be lined up for display like so many artifacts in a museum (Boas 1940). He thus prompts us to ask a very unsettling question: Once we begin to strip away the contextual entanglements from the words in the way that dictionaries do, what is left of the communities that created them?

Perhaps nothing, and perhaps that is the point. Arjun's notebooks are a shrine to translation and translatability—tabulating, ritualizing, and giving presence to contextual meanings and arbitrary codes. This is a deeply personal celebration of and solution to the problem of equivalence that the experience of words in context sometimes serves to hide. Arjun has honed a technique of mind that displays the association of form and intention in its barest state. In so doing, he is manipulating the *sense* of language. He is manipulating, in other words, exactly the thing that those around him believe he cannot even perceive. If Arjun's language is *nakali* to his family because of its ostensible transparency, theirs can just as easily be dismissed for its displacement to something no more complex than a spreadsheet. He is trivializing spoken language by making it look easy. He is, in this regard, making their words *senseless* in exactly the way they assume him to be.

Paradoxically, what makes Arjun unknowable to his family is just how easily he is known. Because nothing he does would seem to require explanation, everything about him that is not immediately available to the senses dissolves into inconsequentiality. His family members do not experience as present the entanglements that make him a social being, and because of these nonperceptions Arjun is caught in a cage of transparency. The things that those around him fail to see define the limits of everything that is possible, and these patterns of possibility and impossibility carve deep grooves of habit that circumscribe his capacity for effective social action. In these terms, fundamental categories like agency, meaning, coherence, intention, and commensurability should be understood not as already existing things for Arjun's family to recognize but rather as the emergent phenomenological consequences of their culturally particular way of *seeing* him.

To these ends, *sense* is a nuanced intuition about how social relationships inhabit things. It's a theory of being with rich texture but also remarkable blind-spots. Arjun—as a consequence of who he is—must navigate the landscape these blind-spots create. In the rest of this book, I will argue that his sensitivities to these dynamics are fundamentally characteristic of deaf cultural practices in hearing Nepal. Specifically, as a deaf man in a nondeaf household, Arjun has cultivated a nuanced attention to the contours of what the hearing do and don't perceive in the world around them. He understands how hearing people engage things that are neither present through form nor available to the senses, and he uses these understandings to foreground social processes that more often than not are simply taken for granted. Arjun's dictionary, for example, is most powerful for its capacity to engineer an experience of both *sense* and *senselessness* in those who use it: words may appear naturally as meanings, behaviors may appear naturally as intentions, and things may appear naturally as causes or effects. But there is nothing inevitable about how any of this plays out. Our intuitions of *sense* entangle people, things, and intentions together, but the particular ways by which this happens end up motivated less by the world as it is than by the culturally embedded ways in which we choose to populate it with vessels of attention. In constructing a universal phrasebook for his family to encounter, Arjun is demonstrating his own radical way of attending to the social nature of things.

By refusing to resolve himself coherently before hearing ways of seeing, I think Arjun offers us an unusual answer to a very familiar deaf dilemma: Is it possible, ultimately, for deaf organizations of *sense* to persist in hearing worlds? Can hearing things act as vessels of deaf forms of value? To see these dimensions of Arjun's dictionary effectively, we need a better way to theorize the problem of *sense*, reorienting our ethnographic engagements around the problem of presence and distinction. How is it that social actors are able to evaluate apparently similar facts, acts, and things as equivalent or not on the basis of the histories of their production? What makes a senseful thing different from a seemingly identical senseless one? These tensions, I will argue, underpin the high stakes of cultural difference, and in this book my primary aim is to share the remarkable insights that people like Arjun bring to them. By intervening in how these tensions unfold for his family, he is revealing—to those who know how to see it—an account of what it means to be deaf in hearing Nepal.

CHAPTER 2

Intelligible worlds

Theoretically, we are aware that the earth revolves, but in practice we do not perceive it; the ground upon which we tread seems not to move, and we live undisturbed.

— Marcel Proust, *In Search of Lost Time*

NECESSARY WORDS

In the previous chapter, I introduced Arjun, a deaf man living in rural Nepal with his hearing family. I described his ambition to create a universal dictionary, and I argued that his life and works are systematically incomprehensible without careful attention to the *sense* of things. "Sense," in this ethnographic context, is a deeply local intuition about the entanglement of material forms by histories of intention. To say that a thing has *sense* is to say that it is experienced by those encountering it as the purposeful extension of people in the course of social interaction. Though Arjun's dictionary was unambiguously useful to his family members as a source of information, they nevertheless experienced it as something without *sense* because they could not perceive in it the traces of Arjun's thinking mind.

The irony, meanwhile, is that Arjun built his dictionary through meticulous attention to exactly the kind of social dynamics that his family members deem him most incapable of understanding. The fact that they could *use* this book without properly *noticing* his place in the history of its creation serves to demonstrate just how much they take for granted about the things they engage with every day. This was, I think, the point. As a deaf man living in hearing worlds, Arjun has cultivated a deep attention to what hearing people do and do not perceive about him, and this attention foregrounds for him dimensions of social phenomena that usually pass by unnoticed. To these deaf sensibilities, what is most notable about dictionaries is just how easily they allow us to forget that words exist as inherently *senseful* things, manifest in context only through complex and particular histories of social interaction. By drawing his family members into the strange world of bare equivalences and contextless meanings that dictionaries imagine, he engineers for them exactly the kind of *senselessness* they ascribe to him.

In this chapter, I will contextualize Arjun's story within a broader frame of Nepali deaf culture, situated at the intersections of deaf political sensibilities and hearing patterns of perception. At these junctures, deaf communities in Nepal have crafted ways to foreground the habits of notice that shape both their own experiences and how they are experienced by the hearing people around them. Any ethnography of deaf Nepal must likewise be sensitive to these dynamics as well. For the task of this book, understanding Arjun and his peers is ultimately a question of knowing how the hearing see. This story, the subject of this chapter, begins in the institutional halls of deaf Kathmandu.

In the spring of 2008, the Kathmandu Association of the Deaf (KAD) invited a small group of language teachers and other allied experts to attend a workshop at its central office. The purpose of this meeting was to assemble a list of "Necessary Words," precisely three hundred basic vocabulary items selected to cover the world's most important everyday things. The aim here was explicitly and expansively polylingual, tied to a number of different ambitions that KAD had for the linguistic proficiencies of the Nepali public: as a benchmark of linguistic competency that could be translated into any language, the list would help hearing people to learn NSL, nonstandard signers to learn officially sanctioned forms, native signers to learn written Nepali, and everyone to learn English. By synchronizing what it means to know a language across modalities and forms, the list's designers hoped to provide (in the words of one particularly enthusiastic language teacher) nothing less than the "planks of a bridge across the chasms of linguistic isolation."

Though the value of this project seemed to go without saying for everyone present, the group quickly found itself mired in controversy as it tried to decide which words, specifically, should be included. Proper nouns were nixed early on in a nod towards economy, and anything that could be replaced effectively by a more general term usually was. One participant suggested "taxi," only to be told that her understanding of taxis as "necessary" revealed in no uncertain terms a deep and dangerous class bias. Religious words and political jargon were complete nonstarters, and even the color spectrum was ultimately reduced to a "good enough" palette of just black, white, and red. Initially, the committee was more tolerant of core edibles like rice, lentils, meat, and eggs, but the mood soured once again when it became clear just how slippery the food slope was: If we were including eggs, why not pomegranates, fried dumplings, and bitter gourds? What about the foods that Madeshis eat but the hill tribes don't, or vice versa? This meeting was taking place at the height of a contentious national election, and the task of determining which things in the world were "necessary" quickly became a proxy for politics. These were old tensions, to be sure. The workshop included a core and periphery of people who had been collaborating together for decades on the institutionalization of NSL, and this shared history charged the meeting with both personal and ideological ambivalences. To the significant extent that claims about language mirror claims about the world, the stakes of how language *ought* to be are inevitably high.

Just as the arguing was starting to turn ugly, however, a deaf teacher from a rural school stood up and proposed a new word: *braille*. Given the tone of the room, I expected her suggestion to be rejected or even ridiculed, but much to my surprise the entire assembly simply nodded in agreement. Without comment or explanation, the word was added to the whiteboard. Just a half-hour earlier, the word "(to) write" had been eliminated for being overly specific, and yet a printing system used exclusively by *the blind* somehow made the cut. My confusion must have been legible on my face, because at this point the woman who proposed the term turned to me and answered the question I hadn't yet asked: "Because everyone thinks we use braille, and *every single day* we have to explain that we don't."

For a variety of material, linguistic, and cultural reasons, deaf people often don't make sense to those around them. They are, to borrow a phrase frequently offered by my hearing informants, "always surprising." The particular contours of this fact vary considerably from context to context, but the constant need to *explain* what being deaf does and doesn't mean seems to be the closest thing we can find to an ethnographic universal among all deaf people everywhere: yes, the deaf are able to use language; no, their other senses are not heightened to superhuman levels by the absence of hearing; no, NSL is not derived from Nepali (nor English, nor any other spoken language); no, sign language is not universal; no, signers don't particularly wish that it were; and, no, deaf people do not use braille.

This air of misrecognition is familiar to deaf communities worldwide, but certain demographic facts make the experience of deafness in Nepal especially vulnerable to misinformation. Owing to the relatively high frequency of prenatal and early childhood illnesses, Nepal has an unusually large number of deaf people.[1] Because of the rugged terrain and general lack of infrastructure, only very few of them come into sustained contact with each other. As a population, the deaf are simultaneously ubiquitous and isolated, and these circumstances leave the hearing world especially unbridled in choosing how to know them. In the words of one deaf community leader, "Everybody in Nepal knows one deaf person, but very few know two." A bit of poetic license aside, this claim is broadly accurate, and I think it characterizes something fundamental about how deaf people are known in hearing places.

For many hearing people, a single deaf neighbor, cousin, or childhood playmate must constitute both the rule and the exception of deafness, shaping the broader class in generalities while at the same time providing the material to defy it in specifics. Over and over again and often unsolicited, the hearing people I met would tell me that they did know one deaf person from back in the village, but—and this was the important part—he or she was completely unlike other deaf people. Usually, this would follow with an anecdote meant to illustrate facility, intelligence, or good conduct in some form or another. These stories were invariably framed as encounters with the unexpected, but—where the deaf are concerned—the unexpected is unusually common. This paradox is so familiar as an experience that it has even warranted a dedicated turn of phrase: *lāṭo po bāṭho*, "the dummy [dumb-y] was actually smart!"

In this world composed of exceptions, the question of generalities becomes a powerful open space. What this speculative freedom has produced in Nepal (and elsewhere, for that matter) is a range of just-so stories about the nature of language and personhood that feature the deaf prominently. Tales about feral

---

1.   Nepal has a deaf population that is roughly equivalent in absolute size to that of the
      United States, a country with ten times the population (Mitchell 2005).

children, for example, came up surprisingly often in my conversations with the hearing about deafness. Though my informants would usually balk when I asked them to make the connection explicit, they always noted that children raised in the wilderness *also* couldn't speak. Many added that this separation from language presented us with a rare opportunity to see what people would be like in the absence of law, religion, education, family, or whatever other basis of social organization seemed most important to them at the time. These grand speculations about the nature of human beings without language—more than any direct experience with actual deaf people—often served as the starting point for elaborate descriptions of what deaf people, in general, are like.

Deaf lives are lived in predominantly hearing worlds, but hearing worlds are often unkind to deaf ways of being. Though this unkindness is sometimes a matter of overt cruelty, more frequently it takes the shape of an inability to perceive deaf value. When you're deaf, it's just harder than it would otherwise be to get people to take you seriously. Arjun's experiences are certainly extreme in this regard, but the constraints imposed by hearing assumptions remain a deep and daily part of all deaf experience. As one deaf man in his mid-thirties put it while recounting for me the challenges that deaf people face, "Good workers have trouble finding jobs, attractive people have trouble finding dates, and the rich even have trouble spending their money." When I asked him to elaborate on this last point, he explained:

> Whenever I go buy something expensive at one of the stores on Durbar Marg [a high-end shopping district], the sales clerks are always confused. Their jaws drop when I pull out a big stack of 1,000 rupee notes to pay. They're like, where'd you get that money? So I hand them my business card, and they see it's from [a well-known company]. I point to my name, next to the title "Director," and I point to myself. They look at the card, then they look at me, then back at the card, then back at me. Back and forth. They don't know what to say. They're afraid to sell me anything because they think their boss will yell at them. So, while they stare, I smile, I put the money I owe on the counter, I take whatever I bought, and I leave.

In this environment of quiet erasure, it is perhaps no surprise that the deaf often take great pleasure in watching the hearing stumble through their own misconceptions. This might be where braille comes in. There is something very satisfying, at any rate, about imagining the hearing as they contemplate the deafness of blind things. The image of people who cannot hear staring intently at something made for people who cannot see is powerfully absurd, and the basic misunderstanding it reveals goes a long way to discredit hearing assessments of deaf competencies. Braille might be, in other words, an opportunity to showcase hearing ignorance.

When I proposed an interpretation along these lines to some of the teachers from the Necessary Words meeting, however, they agreed that I was missing the point entirely. It is indeed funny that hearing people experience braille as a deaf thing, they said, but that is not what makes it a Necessary Word. Rather, in the spaces of hearing misperception, the deaf are often called to act as though absurd things are true, suspending their own patterns of judgment just to be effective in public. These rhythms of misrecognition are something that seems to follow the deaf, and collective lifetimes have taught them to expect it. Absurdity, in other words, is a privilege of the powerful, available only to those who are used to having their intuitions match and shape public reality. At many deaf moments in many deaf lives, *not knowing braille* is itself an important descriptive fact, and in the course of accommodating the hearing across these disjunctions braille *actually* becomes a deaf thing. In any case, as one of the project's authors later suggested to me, isn't the possibility that the deaf and the hearing might talk about braille *together* far more important than the particular deafness or nondeafness of braille as a thing in itself? Perhaps a single shared point of reference is all that's necessary to elaborate an entire world of shared experience. If that's all it takes, why shouldn't that point of reference be braille?

Though I find this explanation convincing on many levels, I am skeptical that braille is really so neutral a thing as merely something to talk about. There is, first and foremost, a question of audiences. KAD was founded to represent the deaf in Kathmandu, but it does so primarily as an interface to a very particular set of national narratives about modernity and development. In this political and historical context, that means asserting deaf difference as part of an aspirational pluralism. All public claims made by KAD about the Necessary Words must be to these ends explicitly and inherently pedagogical, built around hopes for a world in which the hearing and the deaf understand each other more fully. I wonder, however, if the deaf are actually so uniform in their ambitions. Arjun, for example, constructed his dictionary without ever trying to explain what it meant. It contained no reference to NSL, and he showed remarkably little interest in using it to prove to his parents that he was more than they assumed. Even as his notebooks circulated in public, their logic of organization remained private, even covert. In this chapter, I will argue that this tension between public engagements with the hearing and private alignments of value is fundamental to everything we should understand as most central to deaf cultural practices (cf. Bechter 2008). The deaf often want to educate the hearing, to be sure, but just as often they work to populate the hidden corners of hearing worlds with deaf ways of being. To see this tension and how it exists within the Necessary Words project, we must look past the public narrative and into the more particular contours by which braille is experienced by the hearing as something deaf.

One afternoon, several years after the Necessary Words workshop, a group of engineering students arrived at KAD. They had been sent by their college to satisfy a service requirement, and in pursuit of these duties they were looking for an opportunity to build things that would improve the lives of deaf people. The dozen or so KAD members present that day offered a number of suggestions, ranging from strobe-light doorbells and video baby monitors to automatic subtitle systems and watches that vibrate at the sound of car horns. After twenty minutes of back-and-forth through an interpreter, however, the students started showing signs of their bewilderment. Eventually, the youngest-looking of the group spoke up, "We don't really know how to do any of that. We were thinking we could build you some ramps or something." As the words left his mouth, his friends seized with mortification. He registered their response with immediate self-doubt, but it was clear that he didn't understand why they were reacting as they were. For a full five seconds, he searched the room for clues but found instead only deaf faces lighting up with smiles and smirks as the interpreter relayed his message. I don't know what ultimately led him to his answer, but eventually he leaned his head back, took a deep breath, and said softly to himself, "Deaf isn't that kind of disabled."

Indeed, deaf is not that kind of disabled, but—for a few moments, at least—it seemed like it was. The fact that this mistake was even possible shows how strangely generalized intuitions about the nature of disability can become (see especially Sharp and Earle 2002; Ingstad and Whyte 2007). There is no obvious reason to think that the deaf, the blind, the immobile, the cognitively impaired, and the mentally ill should all share a basic experience of the world, and yet "disability" remains somehow a coherent designation in this context. It functions not as a clear or explicit category but rather as a logic of encounter, one conditioned in this case by the demands of a college syllabus. These students came to KAD ostensibly to meet and serve the deaf, but what they encountered instead had less to do with deafness than with their own distinctly modernist intuitions about labor, capacity, obligation, and governance (cf. Davis 1995; Hahn 1997). They wanted to accommodate those who lack, but in the course of actual engagement the particularities of that lack were less present to them than the obligation to meet it.

What this interaction reveals, I think, is the breadth of a gap, one separating what this young engineer *knew* as fact and what he *experienced* as present in front of him. He no doubt understood how ramps engage wheels (with an engineer's precision, no less!), and he could certainly see the deaf people before him moving freely by the power of their own two feet. Nevertheless, ramps at this moment *seemed* to him something intuitively deaf. This intuition was powered not by a lack of knowledge about functions or identities but rather by a distinct structure of attention, shaping what was accessible to him about the world at that moment. To this hearing way of seeing, ramps made *sense*.

It is in these same terms that I would propose to understand braille as a Necessary Word. It is not enough to say that the hearing simply misunderstand braille's form or purpose because—simply—most of them don't. When asked directly, the overwhelming majority can describe it and its mechanics with unhesitating accuracy. Nevertheless, in the course of interaction, braille is attributed to the deaf with surprising ease and frequency. The deafness of braille, like the deafness of ramps, is not a fact of positive knowledge but rather a tacit expectation; it goes without saying, and it evaporates under too direct an analytic gaze. What organizes this space of eyes, sounds, wheels, bumps on paper, and people must be something else, more basic and yet also more elusive.

In this book, I argue that the social circumstances of deaf people in Nepal are shaped by the problem of *intelligibility*. At face value, this is uncontroversial. Deaf people and hearing people use natural languages that occur in fundamentally different material modalities, and it should come as no surprise that they often don't understand each other very well. But, as I will demonstrate, there is far more at stake for the deaf than simply "being understood" as speakers and as subjectivities. Instead, I propose to think about *intelligibility* as a methodological problem, one situated at the intersections of perception and ontology.

As I use the term in this book, *intelligibility* is the quality of being foreground against a background. Things are intelligible when they are experienced by people as fully *present* in the course of social interaction. Things are unintelligible, conversely, when they remain unnoticed, unreferenceable, or lost to the noise. Sometimes, this is a matter of absolutes, and in this chapter we will look closely at how frequently deaf people, practices, and values pass completely unseen though hearing worlds. More often, however, the dynamics of intelligibility are both partial and patterned, built not from total imperception but rather from strange gaps of salience. When the hearing attribute braille to the deaf, for example, they deploy it as a remarkably naked semiotic form, rendering it discursively while not perceiving the functional dimensions most consequentially particular to it. In these moments, braille is encountered not as a technology born from any history of invention nor even as a strategy in the here-and-now for manipulating the senses. It is, instead, a bare solution to a bare problem at moments when neither is really being seen.

Braille is a deaf thing, in other words, because deafness itself is so frequently unintelligible to the hearing. It exists for them not as a particular organization of the senses but instead as an undifferentiated kind of lack, accommodated by ramps, bumps on paper, and strobe-light doorbells equivalently. What drives this intuition is not an absence of knowledge but rather an excess of familiarity, one that allows the hearing to act in the world without ever coming to full awareness of the things closest to them. By foregrounding braille as a Necessary Word, however, the deaf position it as something to be thought about and explained. They make it an object of attention, and in so doing they cause it to become intelligible once again. In the course of this transformation, braille reacquires its own very tactile particularities, establishing a new and fuller presence that forces the hearing to think explicitly about what it means to hear, what it means to see, and what aspects of the world manifest differently to sight and to sound. In these terms, then, braille is a deaf thing because it makes deaf experience something that the hearing must *notice*. It extends the perceptual realities of deaf subject positions onto hearing bodies, and it reveals deafness more fully in context as something embodied, particular, and present. As a Necessary Word, what braille offers the deaf is a basis of engagement with the hearing and their taken-for-granted regimes of expectation.

Though this framing of *intelligibility* draws many parallels to Heidegger's concept of presence-at-hand (*Vorhandenheit*), my interest here is not ontology or phenomenology per se. Instead, my aim is to trace these domains as architectures of intersubjectivity in explicitly ethnographic terms. Consequently, I am less concerned in this book with existential questions than I am with the patterned histories of unnotice that organize encounters in Nepal between deaf and hearing worlds. *Sense*, defined in the previous chapter, illustrates one particular structure of intuition about these dynamics. When Arjun's mother described her son's language notebooks as *senseless*, for example, she was acknowledging that she could not perceive in them the lateral entanglements of social history that should normally accompany these kinds of things. She could not perceive, specifically, Arjun's intentions in making them or the linguistic aptitudes that their making should reveal. These things were there, of course, but they remained for her unseen.

Arjun noticed these gaps in his mother's ability to engage him, and he talked about them frequently. When he did, he would often use the same expression to describe them: *her awareness is only half.* This is a familiar idiom in NSL, though the particularities of its phrasing leave it easily misunderstood. The point here is not that Arjun's mother was relatively more or less cognizant of her son in any absolute terms. No one is ever "fully" aware of anything, of course, and these constraints on human cognition are well understood by philosophers and deaf Nepalis alike. Instead, I think the point Arjun was making is that his mother's way of *seeing* was itself only one side of a dyadic social relationship. Her awareness was only half, in other words, because Arjun's awareness was the *other* half. Worlds are built in the shared spaces of encounter between the deaf and the hearing, but more often than not these worlds are made from deep asymmetries about what is and isn't intelligible in place. To find the deaf, we must first learn to see the contexts and circumstances of these disjunctions.

FINDING THE DEAF

In Kathmandu, deaf people are surprisingly hard to find. In my interviews, hearing residents of the city frequently insisted that they had never actually seen any deaf people there, though they always had stories to tell about a deaf person or two living back in the village. While I don't doubt the sincerity of these claims, it is hard to reconcile them with the actual demographic facts. Nepal is a predominantly rural country, and rural life is often marginal and isolating for the deaf. Like many other stigmatized groups, deaf people have migrated disproportionately to urban areas in search of opportunities and communities that tend not to be forthcoming back home (see Central Bureau of Statistics 2011; World Health Organization 2011; and also Padden and Humphries 1989; Senghas 2003; Lane 2010). As far as raw numbers go, the deaf should be ubiquitous in Kathmandu. The fact that they are not experienced as such illustrates something important about how deaf people do and do not get noticed.

On the city's busy bus system, for example, the ticket collectors I spoke to said they encountered deaf people on virtually every cycle of their routes, and yet the passengers on those same buses could not recall seeing a deaf person on public transit even once. Temple priests at neighborhood shrines repeatedly told me that they couldn't remember the last time a deaf person had come to make offerings, and yet the beggars working outside those same temples could always identify for me numerous deaf regulars by sight. One Kathmandu-born shopkeeper I knew even claimed that he had only ever seen sign language on television, despite the fact that his open-air store sat directly between the city's largest school for the deaf and a major transit hub. Every morning and every evening, literally hundreds of signing children passed through his immediate field of vision, and yet without the four corners of a TV screen he was literally unable to see them. It was only when I sat down with him and pointed at groups of signers walking by that he began to notice what had always been there. Though the deaf may very well be everywhere in Kathmandu, seeing them requires careful alignments of perception (cf. Latour and Woolgar 1986; Stallybrass and White 2007).

This paradox of number and visibility is undoubtedly related to the very fragmented geographies that compose deaf Kathmandu and the very unusual terms by which deaf people constitute a social group. The deaf don't live in or come from any particular place. They don't self-organize in the familiar sites of politics, religion, or trade. They don't usually marry other deaf people, and they only rarely have deaf parents or deaf children. They don't identify themselves through distinctive dress, and nor are they available to identification by the familiar markers of ethnicity, caste, or socioeconomics. When deaf people move in public, they just don't tend to get noticed. As one deaf man put it, invoking the prominent social alignment functions of headwear in Nepal, "There is no such thing as a deaf kind of hat." As a consequence, the deaf—in the most literal sense—are often very hard to see.

Finding deaf Kathmandu thus requires attention to the public intersections of perception and space, and this process lays bare fundamental questions about the nature of disability and difference. Within Nepal's emerging disability activism, for example, the deaf are a prominent and socially leveraged constituency, and yet their participation in this work is unexpectedly controversial. Many in the community will even claim off the record that deaf people do not even understand what it means to be disabled. In the words of one prominent activist:

People see my limp before they see my face. That's all they see. When I walk through *Asan Tol* [a particularly crowded market], every mother, father, sister, brother, and child sees me from all the way across the square. Even the grandmothers and grandfathers see me with their weak and failing eyes. I am always being seen, and the deaf don't understand this.

Leaving questions of "authentic" disability aside, this observation about how the deaf get seen is something that deaf people themselves attest to. They tend to pass very easily through hearing worlds, forced to appear deaf only in contexts of intimacy, close contact, or focus (cf. Ablon 1990; Susman 1994; Shuttleworth 2004). The hearing might certainly notice when deaf people do not respond to audible calls, for example, but this act of calling itself requires an already individuated attention at odds with the anonymity of passage through public space (Warner 1990, 1993; Habermas 1991; but also Gal and Woolard 1995). In more public settings, the deaf blend in with the environment in ways that limps, scars, religious paraphernalia, and markers of race and caste simply don't.

Precisely because the deaf are so hard to find, however, knowing how to find them can itself serve as a mechanism of inclusion for the initiated. In crowded places, signers are remarkably good at spotting other deaf people, and in my interviews they frequently characterized this ability as a distinctly deaf skill (see Bahan 2009; and also Babb 1981). In NSL, this so-called "deafdar" (see Swinbourne 2015) is realized as a satellite dish-shaped hand that sweeps across the horizon of view, pulsing as it passes other deaf signers. As these pings de-anonymize the crowd, the act of noticing others is cast as a palpable sensation. It is worth noting, however, that this radar can malfunction, too. When Nepali signers return from abroad, for example, they will sometimes talk about how exhausting foreign travel is made by the unselfconscious habits of gesture that accompany hearing speech. In one's home country, signers learn to tune out these distractions, but the intuitions that allow them to do so are built from years of encounter with particular patterns of movement. In other contexts, the deaf find themselves suddenly miscalibrated. All of this visual noise then ceases to remain in the background, and hearing gesture starts to look like sign. Seeing the deaf, at these moments, requires knowing how to leave everything else unseen.

In some circles, these dynamics of notice even serve as the basis of a game. In a restaurant or other noisy but enclosed public space, signers will sometimes compete against each other to see how long they can sign before the hearing people around them start to notice. There is a delicate art to achieving this end, and the group of college-aged men who first explained it to me took obvious pride in its mastery. When the game is being played skillfully, the hearing are drawn in *gradually*. They glance over from their tables intermittently, as if they had caught sight of something out of the corner of their eye. Signing is made *almost* present, but never quite enough to be realized as such. To accomplish this effect, players must carefully modulate their movements to sit right at the cusp of conspicuousness: they exaggerate the oral features of NSL and understate its manual components[2] in order to tiptoe at the threshold of what those around them are able to tune out as they enjoy a meal. The players drag this on for as long as they can or as long as they find entertaining, gradually crescendoing their understated movements into an almost wild flailing of arms. Eventually, it is all just too conspicuous not to notice. When the hearing finally *see* sign language, the deaf have revealed themselves, and the game is over.

Though this all may seem an odd sort of prank, it works surprisingly well. When the hearing ultimately recognize signing at the table across from them, their reactions often verge on slapstick: a physical jolt at the end of a long, blank stare or an expression of awkwardness punctuating a direct but inattentive gaze. I once saw an unwitting participant even spill an entire glass of water on herself because she was so startled when she finally noticed the signers sitting right in front of her. It is fun to watch as people experience this transformation in their attentions, and it takes great skill to manipulate how and when they do. As with many interaction genres favored by the socially marginal, the game works by putting powerful people into situations that make them look and feel ridiculous (Bakhtin [1965] 1984; Stallybrass and White 1986). As a sensory phenomenon, this game can be very unsettling. Signing accumulates in the background as an unnameable impression without ever fully manifesting itself (a "psycho-geography," as per Debord [1955] 2008; Sadler 1999). Ultimately, the hearing are embarrassed to realize that they have been staring, but they generally don't

---

2.   These facts of notice are motivated by distinctly Nepali habits of language, including and especially the oral features of signing and the gestural features of speaking. In short, there is a greater perceptual continuity between signed and spoken languages than might be expected both in Nepal and elsewhere. Like in many signing communities, Nepali signers often incorporate morpheme mouthing and other oral organizations into the signing stream (Lucas and Valli 1992; Ebbinghaus and Hessmann 1996). Conversely, though hearing gesture is organized in very different structural terms than signing proper, there are extensive and nuanced formal continuities between the two (Kendon 2004; Goldin-Meadow 2005a; McNeill 2005).

realize that they are staring until they realize that they are staring at *something*. Sign language comes as a surprise in this regard, but the surprise is the fact that it has been there all along.

What this game demonstrates is thus a basic asymmetry of knowledge and sensitivity: when deaf people and hearing people encounter each other in public space, they do not do so on equal terms. Instead, they relate to each other on the basis of very different extents of attention paid to how the other perceives. One deaf participant, for example, compared the effects of the game to what he sees hearing people do when searching for the source of a sound they cannot recognize:

> You see them focused, looking at their work and then suddenly they hear it and they look around for what they heard. They heard it but they can't find it. They don't even know what it is or where it is. They know it is there, maybe. This game is like that.

What this description reveals is a nuanced attention to sound, experienced by the deaf not as an acoustic phenomenon but rather more deftly as the visual effects of its presence on the hearing. Hearing people, conversely, remain unable to see sign language even with wholly functioning eyes. That juxtaposition is the spirit of the game. There is just something very satisfying about revealing how profoundly unaware the hearing can be about the world immediately around them. When deaf people play this game together, they participate in an especially sense-based orientation to the problem of community. They orient deaf attention to the penumbras of hearing perception, and in so doing they cultivate a sensitivity to the ways in which deaf things come to be present in hearing worlds.

In this same spirit of critical reflection on the basis of community, Stefan Helmreich and Michele Friedner accomplish something tremendously important for ethnographic engagements with deaf perception in their essay "Sound Studies Meets Deaf Studies" (Helmreich and Friedner 2015). As they astutely observe, the visual entanglements of deaf lives have served as an old and important domain of research, but this focus has been marked by a tendency to neglect the nuanced ways in which sound becomes present to deaf people precisely through nonhearing. They illustrate this principle with a joke famous in American deaf communities: In the middle of the night, a young deaf man leaves the motel room where he and his wife are staying to fetch something from their car. When he gets there, he realizes he has forgotten his room number. After a short bout of panic, an idea occurs to him. He blasts his car horn for a full minute, and then watches carefully as every room lights up except one. He returns to the room still dark, where his sleeping wife waits. This sensitivity to the perceptions of others, which Helmreich and Friedner call "inferred sounds," is basic to deaf public sensibilities in Nepal, and what it reveals is the inextricably *social* nature of perceptual experience. Absence can be no mere absence when others encounter it as something there.

In the rest of this book, I will characterize the domain of these engagements as a landscape of perception, organized by what I have reluctantly called "deaf activism." This is a label of convenience more than precision, lumping together the loosely amalgamated set of people, institutions, discourses, ambitions, and projects that at least occasionally participate in deaf social and political advocacy in the context of a Nepali public. Because deaf activism is concerned chiefly with the fact of deaf people in a predominantly nondeaf world, the ebbs and flows of salience that make deaf social forms *present* to be noticed by the hearing are of basic importance. These circumstances reveal a methodological dilemma, however. To articulate deaf activism as a discursive orientation, as has generally been done, is to unintentionally but inevitably erase the transactional histories of intelligibility that populate hearing worlds with deaf things. It is a mistake, in other words, to presume that the deaf and the hearing engage over an equivalent field of perceivable objects because it is a field that they themselves are making—differently—in real time. As a consequence, the existence of deaf things cannot be reduced to a theoretically abstract hypostasis but instead must be revealed in context through explicitly ethnographic forms of descriptive attention. To see something, to talk about something, to use something, or to engage something all depend on a prior fact of *being* in social place. Where the deaf are concerned, however, this fact of being in place is conditioned by histories and intuitions that must never be taken for granted. Instead, it is these contours of being and hearing that most profoundly shape deaf lives.

DEAF GEOGRAPHIES

If there is to be an anthropology of the deaf, there must necessarily be something about the deaf that is *specific*. There must be, in other words, a content of form and a configuration of flow that characterize deaf people and deaf ways of being in the world. We must be able to talk about social facts that are deaf but not nondeaf, and we must be able to argue that seeing deaf cultural specificity is important because it is only in these terms that deaf lives can be made intelligible to hearing ethnographers. To precisely this end, it has long been the intervention of anthropology to postulate the existence of practices, forms, and ideas whose coherence cannot be established in individuals but only in groups, without which the happenings of the world would remain inscrutable and seemingly unmotivated. In this sense and for the purposes of this book, culture is the last stand, the architecture of coherences that is necessary because it is irreducible to other things.

In the American context, the question of deaf culture has been articulated primarily around a politics of identity and valorization, located especially in deaf schools and clubs. This history has even yielded a widely adopted typographic convention: in much of the literature, the word "deaf" is used to refer to individuals with an audiological disability, while the capitalized form "Deaf" is reserved for the overlapping but not identical group of people identifying as an ethnolinguistic minority. Though this distinction has served as an important basis of organization in international d/Deaf activism, the particularities of its realization are striking. Orthographic capitalization—the contrast between <d> and <D>—isn't present in either speech or sign, and nor is it a distinction made in Nepali's Devanagari script. It is an opposition of categories that manifests on the printed page but collapses everywhere else. Though this book remains agnostic about the theoretical utility of d/Deaf distinctions in the American context, they remain broadly foreign to Nepal. Here, neither the fonts nor the ideologies make a clear separation between audiological conditions and cultural identities. Finding the logic and substance of deaf cultural difference instead demands a more locally organized approach.

The contours of these local organizations were made especially clear to me early in my fieldwork by a famously severe leader of the Kathmandu deaf scene. We were attending an all-deaf party at a public restaurant, and I commented that it was nice to see a place entirely overtaken by signers. Noticing my enthusiastic note taking, she responded critically: "This isn't a deaf experience. When the party finishes and all these people try to explain where they live to taxi drivers . . . *that* will be a deaf experience." She then waited for me to put my notebook back in my bag, nodding approvingly when I did. Even by this point just a few months into my research, our interactions had taken on a strong pattern in these terms. Though she was always very generous with her time, she made no secret of the fact that she doubted my ability to understand and describe deaf experiences coherently. At this moment especially, I wondered seriously if she was right.

At one level, I grasped what she was saying immediately: she was drawing my attention to the problem of place names. In the intermodal realm of speech/sign that deaf people occupy, places are notoriously stubborn referents. As architectures of pure convention, they simply don't translate very well across the articulatory differences of speaking and signing. Imagine trying to communicate the idea of "Cleveland" to a stranger, for example, without using the word itself. In order to reference proper nouns across these gaps of linguistic modality, participants usually need either extensive shared knowledge or a formal convention of equivalence making. Neither of these things can be counted on in the brief moments that pass between hearing taxi drivers and deaf passengers. Nevertheless, however difficult it might be to render in visual form a thing known by a spoken name, being able to cross these chasms of representation effectively is something that deaf people are called to do every day.

This, however, is only part of the answer, and the remainder took me much longer to understand. As the party ended, the deaf people in attendance began to filter back into the anonymity of the city. I approached a friend to clarify further what made riding taxis such a deaf thing. He explained: "You know a lot of deaf people, and you are at KAD every single day. You go there to meet deaf people, and your signing is getting better. But, when *we* go to KAD, we don't even feel deaf. Everybody signs, and deafness evaporates. Then, we go home." His emphasis here landed squarely on the word "home," a place for him and many others that is entirely hearing. I was being told, in other words, that I had misunderstood the geographic dimensions of deaf experience. I had conceptualized the party as an exemplary deaf space, but this search for exemplification was itself entirely missing the point. Deaf people are most deaf not when they congregate together and cease to feel deaf but instead when they cross the thresholds that separate deaf and nondeaf worlds. To seek out purely deaf contexts as constituting that which is most essential about deaf lives is to forget how much effort goes into making deaf communities appear and disappear every day. I was mistaking presences for things and networked relations for absences. This is, in other words, an error born from faulty intuitions about when and for whom the most deeply lived dimensions of deafness are intelligible. Because deaf lives are lived in the complex intersections of an overwhelmingly hearing world, the deaf are least deaf precisely where they are the most typical. What this structures is

an intrinsically ethnographic problem. Finding deaf Kathmandu requires attention to hidden dynamics of geography.

As advocates in disability studies have long asserted, social categories can
never escape their own material conditions of possibility (Cohen 1998; Paterson
and Hughes 1999; Russell 2002). For the deaf, this fact is rooted in the very
pressing but often unnoticed preconditions of their own social contiguity.
Though sound and sight are the most obvious dimensions of deaf difference, the
unique relationship that deaf people have with the space is perhaps even more
important. The fieldwork for this book was conducted chiefly with self-identi-
fied speakers of NSL, a young but fully robust language with approximately five
thousand fluent users.[3] Though this community of speakers is growing quickly,
it constitutes only a small fraction of the approximately two hundred and fifty
thousand to one million deaf people who live in Nepal.[4] As discussed earlier
in this chapter, most deaf people are born into households without other deaf
members, and their roughly even distribution across the country means that
there are few localities with more than just a few deaf people in them. As a consequence, many deaf people in Nepal do not know other deaf people, and some
do not even know that there *are* other deaf people. The deaf are a scattered lot,
and the consequences of this scattering fundamentally shape how the hearing
(including hearing ethnographers) do and do not see them.

The linguistic dimensions of this organization in space are especially critical.
If there is a single social practice that creates readily perceivable categories of
people in the world, it is the use of a language that is known to some but not
to others. The idea that language can motivate, instantiate, and make possible
culturally distinct ways of being developed in anthropology in tandem with the
idea of culture itself (Herder [1772] 2002; Sapir 1921; Bauman 2003). Likewise, it is no coincidence that most children in Nepal are socialized into the

---

3.   This tally is extraordinarily complicated, for reasons discussed extensively in
     chapters 3, 4, and 5. For the moment, however, I offer the number five thousand
     because it is the one frequently cited by deaf people themselves and because it
     roughly characterizes the scope of a core speech community. There is a massive and
     very important periphery to that core of five thousand, and counting that periphery
     in coherent ways is deeply problematic.

4.   Estimates of this number vary considerably but typically converge somewhere near
     three hundred thousand people who were either born deaf or became deaf before
     learning language, or approximately one percent of the country's population (Little
     et al. 1993).

languages of their immediate kin because, simply, those are the people who are there to do it. Deaf communities, however, are organized in very different terms. Because the deaf don't live in any particular place, because they don't generally have deaf parents or deaf children, and because they don't spend a majority of their time with other deaf people, it is decidedly unexpected that they should have a language of their own. Nevertheless, an increasing number of them do. In contrast to nearly everyone else in the world, however, signers live amidst families who don't share their language and apart from friends who do. NSL, in its most everyday realizations, is a language spoken by people who must leave home to do it.

When deaf people in Kathmandu leave home, they come disproportionately to a half-mile stretch of road between the prime minister's residence in Baluwatar and the Jain temple in Gyaneshwor. This road is officially called "Thirbam Sadak," but relatively few people actually know that. It is not that this information is especially hard to come by, and the recent campaign by the post office to mark every permanent building with a numbered street address has made the task even easier. Nevertheless, the name "Thirbam Sadak" just doesn't come up very often. It doesn't seem to be something people have much use for in conversations about the landscape. Though roads and roadlessness are prominent themes in Nepali public discourses on underdevelopment, people only rarely talk about *particular* roads by name.

Instead, Nepal's urban geography is organized on very different principles. When giving directions, locals tend to use named intersections and other radially bounded features as landmarks. Even prominent businesses and government offices will often publish their locations as "fifty meters south of the Gairidhara petrol pump" or "across from the *pipal* tree in Maitidevi." On the rare occasion that an actual strip of dirt and pavement needs identification, it will usually be referenced in descriptive and contextual language: "the road to the bus park," "the winding road we walked on yesterday," or simply "the road uphill from here." This way of talking about roads is *deictic*: it identifies an object of reference not with a fixed, conventional name like the ones given to people, colors, or types of fruit but rather by cues elaborated in context from a foundation of shared knowledge. Telling a taxi driver to take "the road past my youngest brother's old house," for example, is deictic because it requires everyone involved to know who my youngest brother is and where he used to live. To this way of seeing, roads are not ready-made objects but rather something assembled as needed and according to whatever principles are most ready at hand.

There is even a widely circulated (though incorrect) rumor that U2's hit song "Where the Streets Have No Name" was written about Kathmandu. Among the class of bewildered tourists for whom this account is particularly popular, the lack of names is meant to suggest a lack of coherence or perspective. Of course, if a Nepali pop group were to write a song about Chicago as the place "Where the Intersections Have No Names," they would be technically correct but also missing the point. In Nepal, streets don't have names because they don't need them.[5] These are things experienced as convergences, and to transform them into fixed terms likewise feels clumsy, technical, and strange. It forces an alien and unintuitive logic of categories onto the landscape, leaving the world awkward for those who inhabit it. Intersections are things, and thus they have names. Roads, however, are merely the spaces that pass through them.

Though Thirbam Sadak is tenuous as a thing in the world, it is nevertheless the best place to find the deaf in Kathmandu because it is here at this convergence of spatial logics that hundreds of deaf people congregate every day. This corridor connects several of the city's most important deaf institutions, and here more than anywhere else the deaf come to socialize, work, and play.

The most familiar of these deaf institutions is KAD, the organization described earlier in this chapter as responsible for the Necessary Words project. KAD was formed in 1980 by the first generation of graduates from Nepal's first school for the deaf. As part of its broadly conceived mission to improve the lives of deaf people in the city, KAD serves a variety of functions: it is a meeting space for social and political workshops, a classroom for language and skills training, a reception point for foreign deaf tourists passing through the city, and—most importantly, perhaps—a social club. Every afternoon and Friday afternoons in particular, the space fills beyond its reasonable capacity with a cross-section of demographics otherwise unlikely to interact in Nepal: this includes the rich and the poor, the young and the old, men and women, high castes and low castes,

---

5.   There are interesting exceptions to this, such as Ring Road, the East–West Highway, Durbar Marg, and New Road. What is most striking about these exceptions, however, is that they were *meant* to feel exceptional. Durbar Marg is the stretch of road that leads to the Royal Palace. Both New Road and the East–West Highway were designed as ambitious public works projects to showcase connection and transit as features of modernity and development. Kathmandu's Ring Road is less significant as a route than as a boundary, conceptually separating the core of the city from its growing periphery. The city's increasingly popular gated residential colonies have begun to name their streets as well, though here the ambition to reconceptualize the use of urban space is both explicit and integral to their marketing.

and all manner of other people, all deaf. Here more than any place else, deaf people come to be among the deaf: to talk, to plan, to seek help and to offer it, or simply to be in a place where being deaf is unremarkable. This is where deaf people come when they first migrate into the city from the rural periphery, often without money, prospects, or formal language. This is where interpreters get their certifications and where young deaf leaders cut their political teeth. This is also where people come just because the electricity is out at home or because there's nothing good on TV. If a group of deaf people in Kathmandu decide to do something together, they will probably do it at KAD.

A short walk up the road is the Nepal National Federation of the Deaf and Hard of Hearing (NFDH),[6] founded in 1995 to serve a more expressly political role as a national umbrella organization. Over the past three decades, deaf signers have formed dozens of regional clubs in Nepal on the model of KAD, and the NFDH exists to unify and standardize these local outlets, facilitating communication among them and offering a single interface for contact to the various deaf, disability, and development organizations around the world. The environment here reflects the NFDH's ambitions to be something very different from the clubs that it oversees. At KAD, the visual space is dominated by a relentless and rattling noise of motion; this is the din of a dozen simultaneous conversations, silent to hearing outsiders but cacophonous to the familiar. The NFDH, in contrast, has cultivated a more still atmosphere. The chief activities here are visually inconspicuous, mediated by stacks of paperwork and computer screens that do not communicate across a visual distance. As a place organized around written documents, the NFDH engages tasks less overtly mediated by sign language (or, for that matter, *any* language expressed in real time). In keeping with these aesthetics, the NFDH shows relatively little tolerance for casual socializing during office hours. Though individual visitors will often linger in the front room to drink tea and read newspapers long after any ostensible purpose for being there has passed, members of the hired staff and elected board will frequently dismiss the unnecessary and the unwelcome with a simple admonition: "There's work."

---

6. In 2012, the NFDH underwent a restructuring, and most of its work is now carried out under the name "National Federation of the Deaf Nepal." I will continue to refer to the NFDH, however, as that was the institution operating during the majority of this book's fieldwork.

However differently KAD and the NFDH constitute the aesthetics of the deaf community in Nepal, both trace their histories to a third principal institution. The Naxal School for the Deaf is Nepal's oldest organization dedicated to the deaf, and it is the only one administered by the hearing. It sits five minutes by foot from KAD and ten from the NFDH, immediately across from the police headquarters in a nineteenth-century palace compound that it shares with the city's largest orphanage and the national museum of art. It was here in 1967, in drafty dormitories and palatial gardens converted to playgrounds, that deaf people started doing a mundane but transformative thing for the very first time in any sustained way: they started meeting each other. It was here that the idiosyncratic and ad hoc gestural systems used by deaf people everywhere began to coalesce into the conventional language that is now recognized as NSL (cf. Senghas 2004; Sandler et al. 2005; Brentari et al. 2012). The current leadership of deaf Nepal is drawn predominantly from the Naxal School's first few classes, and its burgeoning movements of young signers are composed largely of the school's current students and recent graduates.

This historical legacy is carried forward alongside a contemporary ambivalence, however, one centered on the question of sign language. If the community of five thousand or so deaf activists who are the subject of this book agree on a single thing, it is this: sign language is good; all deaf people should learn it, and more hearing people should, too. In the United States and Europe, the role and value of sign has been deeply controversial (Sacks 1989; Bauman 2008). With the rise of cochlear implants and other prosthetic technologies, questions about signing and deaf education have come to be mired in broader debates about the value of difference and disability in civil society (Sparrow 2005). In Nepal, however, where a single cochlear implant costs more than an average individual's lifetime income, where there are only a small handful of professional audiologists for a deaf population in the hundreds of thousands, and where questions of difference take on very different cultural orientations, these debates are less immediately present. There is in Nepal very little opposition to sign. Nevertheless, many of the hearing teaching staff at the Naxal School were trained in so-called "oralist methods" at the Clarke School for the Deaf in Massachusetts, and as a part of these methods the school for many years banned sign language outright. But, as has happened countless times before around the world, the children at the Naxal School signed anyway, and in so doing they laid the structural foundation for what is now NSL. Amidst these ambivalences of history, the Naxal School is firmly anchored in deaf narratives for its unifying role but also widely criticized for its alignment with hearing values.

Numerous other deaf organizations have risen and fallen over the years, hazard to irregular cycles of funding, personal politics, and need. Though these institutions establish in Kathmandu a very tangible presence of deaf space, this bricks-and-mortar role is itself ultimately secondary to a more general and largely unspecified history of deaf interaction and contact. To track deaf people as they go about their day is to follow them between these three public spaces and their countless private ones. At any given time, dozens to hundreds of deaf signers fill the long and narrow corridor of Thirbam Sadak in the work of being deaf, and for this reason it is the street itself that plays perhaps the most basic role in constituting the geography of deaf Kathmandu. In a very literal sense, the deaf people who come to Thirbam Sadak spend most of their time in passage, moving from one organization to another or simply lingering at some nonplace in the middle. Deaf teenagers spend hours at the neighborhood's many *cold stores* smoking cigarettes and drinking sweet tea. Deaf office peons flit between stationary shops looking for carbon paper, the right color of stamp pad, or a working photocopier. Deaf friends meet in coffee shops before or after institutional events, and deaf couples flee the oppressive intimacy of KAD just to walk up and down the street in relative anonymity.

Mobile phone shops, in particular, tend to draw deaf crowds. Though the rise and spread of wireless communication networks has had broad implications across the country, it is hard to overstate the transformations they have brought to deaf communities. For the hearing, the mobile phone made interpersonal communication a private act: instead of using the public booth at the nearby general store, individuals now used personally designated numbers to contact each other directly. For the deaf, however, the sudden rise of text messaging on mobile handsets was tantamount to the invention of the telephone itself. From a technical standpoint, the history of texting is a history of afterthought. It was added to the technology as a consumer-facing service at the last minute because the cellular signal had some remaining bandwidth undesignated. For the deaf, however, the consequences of this afterthought were new kinds of group possibility. It used to be that to track down another deaf person, you would have your hearing people call their hearing people, or you might just go to KAD and hope that they would show up that day. This was, needless to say, often infuriatingly ineffective. Against this history, cell phones have made it possible for people to talk to each other from within their hearing homes, simultaneously strengthening deaf contiguity while weakening the necessity of individual sites of its manifestation. The mobile phone, in this sense, builds connections but also reintroduces a geographic scattering. This transformation has perhaps undermined to some extent the logistical relevance of the three organizations described above, all while emphasizing the physical and conceptual spaces around them.

Though Thirbam Sadak is not often an intuitive presence for the people who walk it every day, it is nevertheless at this unintuitive locus that the deaf tend to congregate. In this regard, the deaf are both on this road and like this road. They mirror the landscape they occupy, and the landscape mirrors them back. When the deaf are most difficult for the hearing to see, it is because they occupy unfamiliar logics of social contiguity, organized by their unusual alignments of language and kinship. Though they are readily found within the cemented walls of the institutions they have established, it is also in these places that they report feeling least deaf. Across the range of their engagements, the deaf are most easily seen when they most self-consciously resemble the hearing, when the logics of attention, engagement, and history most particularly their own are made least intelligible by the too-easy familiarity of institutional functions and context. Finding the deaf, like finding Thirbam Sadak, requires careful attention to the gap between that which is typical and that which is possible.

Amidst these historical dynamics, many have argued that deaf space is fundamentally convergent in nature (Haualand 2007), built to be assembled, taken apart, and always experienced as temporary occupations of hearing contexts. Critically, however, this process of transformation always leaves a mark. When deaf people move through hearing spaces (as they do across the majority of every day), those spaces remain hearing but can never again be organized solely by hearing principles. Like Hakim Bey's admonition that the surest way to subvert capitalism is to host fleeting orgies in bank lobbies—reminding bankers that their buildings are good for any number of things that they never intended (Bey [1991] 2003)—deaf ways of occupying space demonstrate that not everything hearing must always remain so. When hearing taxis are hired by deaf passengers, for example, they become—for at least a moment—*deaf* taxis, because the men who drive them must undergo the experience of navigating a city mapped not by spoken names but also by deaf logics of description and reference. It is at these points of contact and reorganization that the hearing come briefly to glimpse the geography of deaf worlds. To understand these moments of encounter, however, we must first understand the principles that guide hearing perception. That is the subject of the next section.

THE WORLD IS NOT AS WE THINK IT IS

Though Thirbam Sadak is the center of deaf Kathmandu's many intersecting geographies, it is also a street like many others in the hearing city. It is crowded with shops, most of which sit elevated on thick slabs of concrete as protection against monsoon rains. As in much of the city, the street runs right up against private lots, and thus these bands across the long sides of the road serve as a visible but permeable boundary between public and private space. In this role, they stand as punctuation marks to relentless circuits of movement. Here, women and domestic servants stop to rest as they go about household errands, day laborers unload overfilled *dokos* (bamboo baskets) to make deliveries, homeless children stop to sift through trash piles for recyclables, and teams of unemployed middle-class men wander just to pass the day. As convenient resting places, these steps are filled with people who have stopped in the course of motion. And when people stop on Thirbam Sadak, they are more likely than ever to *see*—in very hearing ways—the deaf people who exist everywhere.

To sit and see is a familiar activity, and among the most prolific sitters-and-seers in Kathmandu are the city's large numbers of unemployed men. One particular group of such men, too old to properly be called young but not yet middle-aged, frequently sat on Thirbam Sadak at a roadside tea shop just across from the deaf school. Unemployed and there because (in their words) they were considered a nuisance everywhere else, they spent most of their afternoons watching people pass on the street. They occupied enough class privilege to have their loiterings tolerated, though the shopkeepers of their parents' generation would often disparage them after they left: "*Naya generation ko problem tehi ho*" (That's the problem with the new generation right there). These criticisms were perhaps meant to tell a story about the character and work ethic of these particular individuals, though a more structural analysis would position them in the penumbra cast by modern expectations of Nepali citizenship (Pigg 1992; Whelpton 2012). After being told for decades that education would provide access to global kinds of productivity and global kinds of wealth, unemployment has come to feel like a quieter kind of failure than would day labor. These are the denizens of a desperately-trying-to-stay-middle class, and their presence on Thirbam Sadak as regular spectators of passage is part of the landscape.

On one particular morning, this tea shop crowd and I sat and watched as students streamed into the local deaf school for class. From the south, we were approached by a familiar figure: a stocky and sun-wrinkled elderly woman who was known for spending her days pacing up and down Thirbam Sadak with a long walking stick. Nobody I talked to knew her name or where she was from, but her distinctive behavior and appearance left her instantly recognizable. She wore a massive bulk of fabrics wound around her body, neck, and head, imbuing her with a radius easily twice that of her underlying form. Some people called her "Kapada Baba"—literally "cloth father." This is a complex and loaded name. In much of South Asia, "Baba" serves as a title of sorts, a simple honorific at times but also a term of address for madmen saints. This latter sense was bolstered by the woman's tendency at unexpected moments to make loud and startling proclamations, often religious in nature. The name suggests an extent of gender transgression as well, motivated perhaps by either the sexless form produced by her abundance of clothing or the vulgar gestures she would sometimes make at gawkers. On this particular day, she was singing loudly. As she moved near us, she came to the attention of one member of the group, and he pursed his lips in a gesture of pointing:

A: *U pani lāṭo ho?* (Is she also *lāṭo* [deaf, derogatory]?)

B: *Bahira, bahira.* (*Bahira, bahira* [deaf, non-derogatory]?)

A: *U pani bahira ho?* (Is she also *bahira?*

C: *Hoina holā.* (Probably not.)

A: *Kina yastai chha, hai?* (Why is she like this?)

B: *Bahira holā.* (She's probably *bahira*)

C: *Hoina. Hāmro peter-ji le bhaneko kurā suninas? Kān sunchhan bhane bahira hũdaina.* (No. Haven't you been listening to what Peter has been saying? If her ears hear then she's not *bahira*.)

B: *Mero ek janā bhāi chha. Yastai chha. Bahira nai ho.* (I have a younger relative. He's like this. And he's *bahira.*)

C: *Bahira ho bhane kasari git gayo, bhana ta?* (If she's *bahira*, why don't you explain how she's singing?)

B: *Bahira holā.* (*Bahira*, probably.)

C: *Sālā.* (Bastard [lit. younger brother-in-law])

They cursed each other for stubbornness, but then proceeded to let the conversation drift back to cooking-gas shortages and the faithlessness of politicians. At the time, early in my research, I found it remarkable that people could wonder if a woman famous for the power of her voice was somehow also deaf. It turns out this is a completely unremarkable possibility, one that has everything to do with the productively imprecise semantics that inhere in the words most often used to identify the deaf in contemporary Nepal: *lāṭo* (lit. "mute/dumb") and *bahira* (lit. "deaf").

The more common of the two terms, *lāṭo*, is in general parlance more evocative than precise. It might certainly refer to someone with an audiological condition (i.e., "a deaf person"), but it needn't necessarily. Anyone, regardless of hearing status, might be *lāṭo* if stubborn enough, stupid enough, or intoxicated enough. *Lāṭo*s are frequently naughty children, unreasonable neighbors, and bad drivers. It is a word with a divided function, one people use when feeling frustrated or mean but also in a more neutral tone to talk about the deaf people in their lives. A man might suggest that his brother is *lāṭo* after an unpleasant interaction, for example, but he will clarify that the man is not *pakkā* (actually) *lāṭo* if further pressed. When wrestled into the unusual task of definitions, Nepalis without fail include the inability to hear or (more precisely) the inability to speak as essential to the term *lāṭo*, and yet instances of the word in everyday talk only rarely pertain to actual ears or actual voices. As a category, then, *lāṭo* pitches deaf people into a fluid domain of literal and metaphorical semantics (Lakoff 1990), much like the English word "dumb." As an attribution attached to people in a particular time and place, *lāṭo* productively conflates the inability to speak with the inability to think. Any distinction between these two possibilities is made only through kinds of attention rarely applied to words in the course of everyday speech.

Such a pattern of usage reflects, among other things, a history of language change. Like all words, *lāṭo* bears with it legacies of its past and anticipations of its future in every instance of utterance (Vološinov [1929] 1986). Etymologically, the word *lāṭo* is derived from a regional dialect where it means simply "maimed, [or] deficient" (Turner 1990). In its contemporary verbal morphology, however, the chief connection is not to any particular nonexperience of sound but rather to the feeling of a limb that has lost sensation. This is a powerful image: a person can be *lāṭo* in the same way that a foot can be asleep. In both cases, we are pointed toward the conflict between a fact of presence and the experience of absence. We might say, in other words, that a *lāṭo* is someone who is there even though it is as if he or she were not.

In recent years, deaf political consciousness has motivated a strong preference for the alternative term, *bahira*, a Sanskrit-derived word that identifies
nothing more and nothing less than an absence of hearing.[7] The purpose of this
reform is very specific: though the use of *lāṭo* to reference the deaf is not usually intended as mean-spirited by the hearing, the word is nevertheless mired in
representations of personhood that are difficult to construe in a positive light.
The power of *bahira* as a publicly correct descriptor is precisely its perceived lack
of connotation.

This same lack of history, however, also makes *bahira* a clumsy word. Outside
of the educated middle class, it's just not something people tend to say. It remains at best clinical and sometimes completely unknown. One man I spoke to
in the far eastern part of the country, for example, became visibly uncomfortable
as he tried to talk about the deafness of his cousin. It seemed that he was aware
that he shouldn't call his relative *lāṭo*, but he was much less certain of any viable
alternatives. As the conversation went on, he found himself caught in acrobatic
circumlocutions, engineered to navigate the fits and starts of this shifting politics of terminology. At one point, he even got up to fetch a bright yellow poster
distributed by a major disability organization in Nepal, contrasting one column
of "words we should say" (including *bahira*) against another column of "words
we shouldn't say" (including *lāṭo*). To the socially marginal, this is a very familiar
politics. The development industry in Nepal has dedicated significant resources
to a broad but concerted awareness campaign. Central to it has been an attempt
to characterize certain forms of denigration and exclusion as a mark of underdevelopment, at home only among backwards-thinking yokels and hillbillies
(Pigg 1996, 2001). As this man later explained to me explicitly, he was eager to
show that he was not, in fact, "backwards," but he became embarrassed when the
new normative terminology began to trip off his tongue. Here, the category of
deafness isn't a particularly ambiguous thing, and yet the terminological terrain
that comes with it is unfamiliar enough to cause speakers to stumble. The deaf
are—very literally in this sense—hard to talk about.

As I was constantly reminded, deaf language is also hard to talk about. Early
in my fieldwork, I tried to write a grammar of NSL. The project was a complete

---

7.   I thus disagree with Erika Hoffmann-Dilloway's suggestion that *bahira* has been
      asserted by activists to invoke an ethnolinguistic model of deafness (Hoffmann-
      Dilloway 2011, 286). Certainly there is a similarity in the way that terminology
      has become a context of activism, but the entailments of each set of categories is
      radically different in the Nepali and American contexts.

and utter failure, and I now realize that several of my closest deaf collaborators had been telling me all along that it would be. Their objections (now better understood) motivate a great deal of the shape and content of this book's next chapter. At the time, however, it seemed odd to me that NSL had its own dictionary but very little documentation of what linguists would call the morphosyntactic structure of the language. I now appreciate that this absence is no accident. Dictionaries and grammars are cultural institutions of the purest kind, and each requires a very particular sensibility about what kind of a *thing* language is. The simple reality is that Euro-American linguistic intuitions only rarely find traction in deaf Nepal. When they do, it is because deaf Nepalis have mobilized them for distinctly Nepali and distinctly deaf theoretical ends. Dictionaries are useful, it would seem, but grammars are harder to assemble in terms coherent to deaf Nepal.

Despite my lack of sophistication, however, my collaborators in Kathmandu were always exceptionally generous with their time. One man I'll call Ujwal in particular subjected himself to more than a hundred hours of videography. I chased him through countless impossible elicitations, each meant to trace the shape of some obscure grammatical constraint or another. How many layers of embedding can a sentence hold? When is tense marking obligatory? Can all verb roots function as nouns, and vice versa? I now know that my questions misconstrued the language so badly as to give off the rhythm of zen koans, but Ujwal always answered as politely as he could. On one particular instance, I was pushing him on the issue of negation scope, and to this end we were talking about things and their opposites. I asked him to construct a sentence about what the opposite of deaf is, and he responded a bit more abruptly than usual:

In Nepal, the opposite of deaf is not "hearing." The opposite of deaf is also not "speaking."[8] The opposite of deaf is "Nepali."

I must have seemed surprised, because at this point he laughed, apologized, and explained that he'd been having a tedious time at home lately. When I asked

---

8. In many signed languages around the world (though notably not NSL), the term used to reference nondeaf people is not "hearing" but rather "speaking," a fact that reflects how disability acquires different kinds of salience for different kinds of subjects.

him to elaborate, he laughed again and pointed out that we had a long day of transcription ahead of us.

We might read Ujwal's statement as an account of opposition, independence, or resentment, but I think it demonstrates instead a remarkably nuanced sensitivity to the way that hearing categories converge on deaf people in time and place. This is a cultural intuition with important methodological consequences, extending well its obvious parallels to the anthropological concept of markedness. By necessity, deaf Nepalis are first and foremost *Nepalis*, not in any sentimental or nationalist sense necessarily but rather to the extent that being Nepali means being entangled in every imaginable axis of difference relevant in Nepal: this is kinship, gender, age, class, caste, ethnicity, politics, and occupation, to name just a few. In these terms, we should wonder what it means to be a deaf woman, a deaf Gurung, or a deaf Brahmin, especially in a context like Nepal where (as Arjun experienced in the first chapter) being deaf serves to push the social entanglements that constitute things like gender, ethnicity, and caste so far into the background. What is it then that fills that space? To Ujwal, I think this question is exactly the point: social overdetermination can produce vast gaps of meaning (Althusser 1969), and the contextually particular ways in which these gaps get filled is what being deaf is all about.

As the conversations about Kapada Baba demonstrate, two people can talk together about something "deaf" without at any moment agreeing or disagreeing about what makes that thing deaf in the first place. The category, in this regard, emerges not as a contentful attribution but instead as a basis for the collaborative experience of something present. The tangle of associations and implications established by deaf things in context are thus made subordinate to a mere fact of *being* in social place. These patterns of experience are made possible by a heavy asymmetry in how the deaf and the hearing encounter each other. Though the deaf talk extensively about the hearing as a class—what they are like, how they should be understood, why they think as they do—hearing people tend to feel hearing *only* when they encounter the deaf. At any other moment, the ubiquity of hearing leaves deafness without an obvious basis of contrast. To call something "deaf" is thus to invoke a presence far more basic and far less precisely specified than any condition of the senses could be. In these moments, the opposite of deaf is not hearing because—for most people most of the time—hearing is so taken for granted that it doesn't warrant an opposite. Except in rare moments of encounter, deaf stands alone. It is the opposite of everything else.

Kapada Baba, likewise, is "deaf" not because she is *actually* deaf but because she is—definitively—not Nepali. As an apparently homeless woman with no obvious family or occupation, she just doesn't fit anyplace. She is, as a consequence, outside. She doesn't have any intelligible entanglements by kinship or civil society, and this distance from all other anchors of reference is what makes her so easy to see as deaf. It is in these terms that we should understand what happened next: Fifteen minutes after our first encounter, just as I was standing up to leave, I nearly collided with Kapada Baba as she was making a second pass back down the road. After regaining her footing, she swung her stick at me and shouted, as if it were a curse, "*Yahi sansār timī le samjheko jasto chhaina!*" (This world is not as you think it is!). After a fierce stare, she continued walking up the road. This was the kind of proclamation Kapada Baba was famous for, and the inhabitants of Thirbam Sadak are usually quick to dismiss them all as raving nonsense. In this case, however, my companions found her words profound. What does it mean to say that the world is not as we think it is? How is it, then? And how does she know? For the men who witnessed it, Kapada Baba's proclamation cast the world in very personal terms. If things are not as they seem, perhaps that explains why it's so hard to find jobs, why food is more expensive than ever, and why the electricity is on for only six hours a day. To accept that things are not as they seem is simultaneously to ask why they are not as they should be. I hoped they would relate these questions back to the ambiguities of deafness they had been discussing earlier, but they did not. Instead, Kapada Baba's presence on Thirbam Sadak served to confirm for them what they had long suspected: that nothing is as it seems.

It is no coincidence that Kapada Baba was an ambiguous deaf person on her first pass down Thirbam Sadak and an oracle of the world's ambiguity on her second. Though she is not deaf in any conventional sense, the circumstances that made her intelligible as such are precisely what caused her proclamation to be experienced as so powerful. By virtue of her appearance and demeanor, she resists easy classification, and she is unencumbered by the more normal kinds of social entanglement. She comes from the outside. She was recognizable as deaf, ultimately, because she made the hearing feel *hearing*. She made them feel, specifically, encumbered by context and history, and in this space of how they relate to her she was made to slip into and out of being deaf with remarkably little conceptual friction. To *call* Kapada Baba "deaf" is thus not best understood as an act of identification. She is not engaged here as a *kind* of person but rather as a *locus* of attention, one that constitutes her as a jointly experienced presence

of something strange. To the deaf, these blank spaces carved by hearing inatten-
tion are familiar, for it is in these spaces that deaf lives are lived.

RAGHAV: BEING TWO THINGS

Raghav Bir Joshi is a prominent member of Kathmandu's deaf community. He
was a student in the first class of the Naxal School for the Deaf, and in the years
since he has served as president of both KAD and the NFDH over multiple
terms. In 2008, he was elected to Nepal's Constituent Assembly, the legislative body convened to draft a new constitution following the deposition of former king Gyanendra Shah. He is also the proprietor a large and well-equipped
printing house, which he manages on property attached to his family home in
the prominent commercial district of Putali Sadak.[9] In these various official and
circumstantial positions, Raghav has come to function broadly as a representative of deaf Kathmandu, and in this capacity even the hearing tend to listen to
what he has to say. He is remarkably good at this job, too. Everyone I talked
to agreed that Raghav is exceptionally talented at persuading the hearing to
reimagine their understandings of what it means to be deaf, and his very public
stature gives him ample opportunity to do so. Through all of this, he has managed to remain both well respected and widely liked by his deaf constituency,
which is no small feat of its own.

As in all political work, Raghav's capacity to stand for Kathmandu's deaf
community is driven by an ambiguous distinction between what is and what
should be. This is never more visible than in the sharp juxtaposition between
Raghav's carefully crafted public persona and the incidental hazards of his private everyday life. As Raghav is a public figure, his daily labors are organized
around the problem of transparency. This begins with the most basic constraints
of communicative efficacy. Unlike most of his political peers, Raghav spends a
considerable part of his day dealing with the logistics of interpreters: vetting
and training them, securing their salaries, making sure they are where he needs
them to be, and shoehorning speeches he plans to deliver in NSL into a spoken

---

9.   Not entirely coincidentally, Putali Sadak happens to be one of the few named streets
     in the city, a fact that reveals its prominence and the prominence of Raghav's family
     for owning significant land there.

Nepali equivalent. Without the aid of these interpreters, he is in the most literal sense unintelligible as a political voice.

In a similar though more abstract vein, Raghav's claim to the Constituent Assembly was framed as an explicit fight against voicelessness. He campaigned on a platform of radical inclusivity with Ramshila Thakur, a well-known advocate for women, and Sunil Babu Pant, the founder of the third-gender[10] advocacy group the Blue Diamond Society. In the wake of nearly three centuries of Hindu monarchy, they argued, the "New Nepal" must embrace not only ethnic diversity but a more encompassing notion of personhood as well. Real change, they said, required "seeing gender, sexuality, and disability in everything."[11] As these three first-time politicians iterated their stump speeches over dozens of rallies leading up to the election, the relationship they saw between voice and visibility became progressively more explicit as a core of their distinctive politics. Nevertheless, these were self-consciously political representations, and to mistake them as constitutive of Raghav's social self is to erase the processes of becoming that situate him as a locus of hearing attention. As soon as he steps off that stage to reenter private life, his intelligibility is once again at stake.

In these terms, following Raghav on a regular day invites the question of what, precisely, is deaf about his life? He invited me to do just that one afternoon a few months after the election. We met at the NFDH office, the only explicitly deaf space in Raghav's travels that day. He had proposed the NFDH as a meeting place for reasons of convenience, but later apologized that this had been a mistake. Immediately upon his arrival, he was drawn in by several office functionaries concerned about "extremely urgent matters" that would require "only a moment." Raghav expressed skepticism about both the importance and brevity of these tasks he was being called to do, but nevertheless his position compelled him to attend to organizational business before anything and everything else.

Though the work accomplished at the NFDH is critical to the well-being of deaf Nepal, it is situated within the quiet functions of everyday office behavior. Everybody here speaks sign language, but—the particularities of signed modalities aside—the structures of communication that organize this place would be remarkably familiar to anyone at home in any of Nepal's countless

---

10. This is a distinctly South Asian concept whose precise implications are well beyond the scope of this book, though it can be linked in rough terms with more global LBGTQ politics.

11. Joshi, personal communication, July 28, 2009.

hearing NGOs. A great deal of time is spent, for example, trying to get the fax machine to work. These patterns of bureaucratic life are motivated by logics of efficacy that largely subsume deaf difference. While writing letters, planning meetings, and engineering grants, Raghav's deafness is inconspicuous except as a fact that legitimates his role in this place. This is perhaps the only context where his intelligibility as a deaf man is never structured by deep asymmetries with the hearing but always assured by his position within a very familiar organizational structure. The surface paradox of deaf sociality, thus, is that the NFDH is simultaneously the most deaf and the least deaf space in Raghav's day (cf. Holmberg 1996).

Paperwork completed, we left the NFDH on Raghav's motorcycle. This was, technically, illegal. The laws have changed in recent years, but at that time deaf people were not allowed to sit for the vehicle licensing exam. This was a controversial policy, and the actual laws on the matter were never entirely clear. Because driving is expensive in Nepal, relatively few deaf people were in any position to test the system. Those who did, however, often framed their choice to drive as a form of civil disobedience.

The Office of Transportation Management, meanwhile, officially maintained that the deaf cannot drive safely because, in the words of one functionary I asked, "their awareness is not one hundred percent." It is the general opinion of deaf Kathmandu that the motivations for this policy are ridiculous, maintained only by people who understand neither being deaf nor the realities of modern traffic. On the busy streets of Kathmandu, they argue, sound is at best unreliable and at worst misleading as an information signal. Deafness, consequently, should be understood really more as an asset than as a liability on the road. Though there is plenty of honking to be heard in the city, the sound is so ubiquitous as to lack signification for anyone but pedestrians as a declaration of vehicular presence. Horns are used primarily not to engage a particular other but rather as a more anonymous form of self-identification, one that screams, "I am here; move out of the way if you'd rather not be run over." Though he cannot himself hear it, Raghav uses the horn on his motorcycle extensively to this precise end.

On the road itself, deaf people are essentially unrecognizable as such amidst the noisy communicative logics of the crowded streets. Given the high stakes that accrue to large metal objects traveling fast in a bustling and unpredictable environment, driving safely requires participation in a complex and precise semiotics of motion and driver intention. In order to not crash, a driver must know how to evaluate what other people intend to do in the immediate future, and this communication happens entirely through nonverbal channels. Traffic in this sense constitutes an interesting geography of perception, hosted amidst blinking turn signals and elaborate inventories of gesture used to negotiate the right-of-way with other motorists. Deaf people understand themselves—rightly in my opinion—as masters of these techniques. Regardless, Raghav was legally prohibited from the road because he is indistinguishable from other motorists as deaf. His passage as hearing is *too* effective to demonstrate to other drivers that he will not be engaged by audible signals. This, ultimately, is precisely the concern that maintains the prohibition of deafness on the road, aligning nonperception against the perceived urgency of legally designated identities. Navigating the streets and these politics, we arrived at Raghav's home without incident (legal or kinetic).

As we parked in the courtyard of his house, Raghav asked if we could stop in the print shop briefly so he could evaluate the proofs for an upcoming job. Inside, the metal plates and rolls of paper were staggeringly loud. Though the print shop's staff was entirely hearing,[12] everyone inside this space is rendered functionally deaf by whirrs and clanks of white noise. In order to get work done in this environment, the printers have invented a narrow but effective system of manual signs to communicate, and they use this system both when Raghav is present and when he isn't. Many of these signs were taken from general NSL, introduced presumably by Raghav but changed enough in their articulation to indicate that they had taken on an independent life among a group of people who were not primarily signers. Other signs were unrelated to NSL (as far as I could tell, at least) and likely indigenous to the printing house itself. When the proofs appeared, this manual signing was replaced entirely by a complex annotation system of ink on paper. This is a space in which Raghav's deafness is structurally unseeable, imposed on even the hearing by a sufficient volume of useless sound. Raghav's employees are not deaf, though that difference between him and them is momentarily collapsed by the crude materialities of heaving steel plates.

---

12. There is an interesting irony to this, which is that European and American print shops were historically staffed by the deaf. For this to be a deaf-owned shop staffed by the hearing, likewise, is a rare kind of comeuppance. I asked Raghav if he knew this, and in response to my question he only smiled politely and remarked that he always finds history interesting.

Work completed, we moved upstairs to the living quarters of the property, where a small gathering was being held for a minor religious festival. At Newar feasts, guests typically eat in shifts, facing inward from around the perimeter of a designated room. When our turn came, we sat and joined. The other attendees were members of Raghav's neighborhood and extended family, all people who had known him since either he or they were children. As a consequence of this familiarity, none of them showed any particular hesitation about communicating with Raghav and me in a pidgin of acquired and ad hoc signs, though notably he was much more able to understand them than I was. The signing was highly idiosyncratic, fluidly shifting between arbitrary fixed signs and real-time pantomimed productivity, with no obvious distinction made for any given bit of speech at any given moment: paper stamped, folded, shoved in a slot—you—thumbs up: "You won the election, good work!" Forked tongue—bandit's mask—glasses—fists pound together—weighing both sides: "Girija and Prachanda [leaders of the Congress and Maoist Parties, respectively] fight constantly. Who will win?" This talk was more heavily influenced by conventionalized lexical items from NSL than is typical for homemade signing systems, a consequence perhaps of Raghav's prominent position in both deaf and hearing circles. None of these signs would necessarily be effective outside of these contexts, but nevertheless they work for Raghav and his family, whose engagement through deafness is overwhelmed by less alien relationships of kinship and intimacy.

As we finished eating, Raghav's elderly aunt called him back to the kitchen. She informed him that the guests were moving through her supply of eggs at a faster clip than she had expected, and she needed him to go to the store to buy some more lest there be nothing for the vegetarians to eat. We headed downstairs and walked to a corner store that Raghav had been visiting since he was a child. The shop owner knows Raghav well and communicates with him as effectively as any family member could. However, at this particular moment, the shop owner was away from his post. In his stead was a young associate of some sort, a son or son-in-law perhaps, who quickly proved himself to be a much less able communicator. This is a familiar reality in deaf Kathmandu: some hearing people are quite adept at improvising communication with the deaf, while others freeze up and fail utterly. As Raghav cycled through various framings and reframings in hopes that he could plant the relatively simple notion of an egg into the mind of his interlocutor, the shopkeeper merely became more and more flustered. More dignified options exhausted, Raghav began flapping his wings, clucking, and dropping round objects from his backside, all while chuckling at the absurdity of it all.

This performance served to embarrass the man behind the counter and to amuse a seemingly impoverished elderly woman who was sheltering herself from the sun under the shop's awning. She had no particular reason to be there, but the sun was hot and shop awnings are a familiar place of congregation for those with nowhere else to be. As the would-be conversation dragged on fitfully, the woman intervened. "These two probably want some candy. Give them some candy, won't you shopkeep?" Raghav looked over at the woman after seeing me do so, and in response she raised her hand in a blessing, muttered a benediction, and shuffled off. Raghav shook his head knowingly. It is the fate of deaf members of parliament, it would seem, to be pitied by even the poorest. Her request for candy, in particular, was telling. In the absence of motivations intelligible to her, I believe she sought to extrapolate Raghav's needs from first principles. Raghav must want sweets because . . . well, people like sweet things. As a deaf person, he was apparently hard to see as wanting anything more socially mediated or complexly instrumental. Meanwhile, the shopkeeper had by this point given up, concluding that communication was impossible, and so he gave himself over to the reductive semiosis of action. He cleared the counter and allowed Raghav to pass into the cloistered backroom where most of the shop's inventory sat. Raghav selected six eggs and placed them into a thin plastic bag. He gave the shopkeeper a large bill, nodded, and walked back outside.

At that moment, Raghav received a series of text messages in quick succession. He read through them and, while waiting on change for his eggs, called over a young boy standing nearby. He instructed the boy to take the eggs up to the feast (with far less difficulty than he'd had with the shopkeeper, notably) and gave him a few rupees for his trouble. He apologized to me for needing to depart abruptly, but he explained that he was needed at the parliament building immediately. The Constituent Assembly was going to be in session soon, and he had to meet with his interpreter to prepare a speech. He was off, in other words, to engineer for the government precisely the intelligibility of voice that remains so uncertain for him when buying eggs.

To spend time with deaf people in their everyday lives is to realize how much of their time is lived in translation. For Raghav, this is both literally and figuratively true. What organizes his experience most strongly is not the fact that store clerks talk to him in patronizing tones nor even the fact that he speaks to parliament as a representative of the people. Rather, it is the fact that he is somehow the kind of person to be patronized by store clerks mere moments before giving speeches in parliament. This, ultimately, is the ethnographic punchline to his story. When hearing people encounter Raghav as deaf, they perceive their encounters as revealing *him* ("he is deaf"). Raghav, however, is more sensitive to how the terms by which others perceive him are conditioned by contingencies of context ("My deafness is very different to the hearing when I buy eggs in shops than when I deliver speeches as a politician"). He is keenly aware, in other words, of how deafness reflects back upon the hearing to reveal their own conditions of notice.

In all of this, Raghav's subjective experience becomes intelligible by making moments of translation appear as totalities, each organized by vast particularities of encounter that are perceived (and often intended to be perceived) as general and whole. The conditions of Raghav's presence at any given moment of engagement are thus both easily mistaken for and fully antithetical to his own subjective self (D. Lewis 2001; Sider 2003). Consequently, though the impulse to locate the deaf in exemplary forms and places is understandable, it is also a serious mistake. Disambiguating Raghav is the surest way *not* to see him. Instead, we might say that Raghav is an exemplary deaf person precisely to the extent that he demonstrates just how difficult it is to find exemplary deaf moments, circumstances, and ideas. Such is the life of a man who is both pitied by the powerless and empowered by an electorate. When I asked Raghav what he made of these contradictions, he merely laughed and told me to get on with my questions.

For anthropologists, the organization of deaf experience builds a descriptive encounter systematically at odds with the reflexes of Euro-American scientific inquiry, articulated as it often is around metaphors of discovery. Anyone who wishes to write about the deaf must of course first set out to find them, but therein lies the rub: the deaf are constantly being found, and their most characteristic social practices are themselves engagements with this process of discovery. Being found, not being found, and being able to effect either of those possibilities at will is a broad and productive space of action in deaf Kathmandu. The classic anthropological ambition to make the foreign intelligible must thus grapple with the fact that deaf people dedicate a great deal of their social labor to making themselves intelligible or not. Engaging with anthropologists writing books, in other words, is a very deaf thing to do. In this regard, the deaf reveal an intrinsic tension between *being* and *perceiving*. They negotiate this tension as a political strategy, and they render the ostensible fact of presence and absence itself as a domain of critical social activity.

Though this theoretical approach is indebted to phenomenology and gestalt psychology, I am positioning intelligibility here as an explicitly *social* phenomenon. How and if deafness becomes intelligible in a given context is the consequence of nuanced cultural particularities, and the manner in which deaf people themselves engage these dynamics constitutes a distinctively deaf set of cultural practices. Consequently, throughout the rest of this book, I will argue for intelligibility not so much as a cognitive fact but as a methodological necessity: to describe the deaf in other terms is to render them incoherent. In this commitment, I echo what Boas observed more than a century ago in his essay "On Alternating Sounds" (Boas 1889): to the significant extent that primary perception is shaped by cultural expectation, imposing the wrong inventory of objects on a phenomenon is tantamount to "blindness." Because the anthropology of the deaf is concerned with a group of people for whom these questions are always at stake, any description of deaf political engagements that begins by presuming a set of already intelligible things is inevitably blind, mistaking moments for wholes and processes for things. Deaf sociality is predicated not on the structure of a particular cultural content but rather on distinctively deaf ways of maneuvering amidst multiple orders of things and a polyphony of possible contents. When we begin by tracking intelligibility itself, a very different and very deaf kind of coherence emerges.

CHAPTER 3

Being transparent

जसरी दृष्टिविहीनहरूले ब्रेल लिपिमा लेखिएका कुरालाई छामेर खर्र पढ्न सक्छन् त्यस्तै गरेर श्रवणविहीन समुदायले पनि सङ्केतलाई सर्र बुझ्न सक्छन् ।

Just as the blind can khrr read things written in braille, so can the deaf community srr understand signs.
– Shilu Sharma, *The Origin, Development, and Structure of Nepali Sign Language*

A HISTORY OF NAMES

I'm not sure how Mahesh found his way to the deaf club. In fact, I don't even know that his name is Mahesh, and odds are that it is not. Anthropologists often have the strange task of assigning fictive names to the people they write about, but for Mahesh even the question of what it means to know a name is unexpectedly complex.

Mahesh arrived at KAD, the Kathmandu Association of the Deaf, with the clothes on his back, enough money for maybe two or three meals, and an aluminum cooking pot filled with root vegetables. He didn't know anyone in Kathmandu. He had been put on a cross-country bus a week earlier by members of his family in the far western part of the country, and he had reached the city's main bus terminal with not much sense of what he would do next. Several days must have passed between Mahesh's arrival in Kathmandu and his appearance at KAD's doorstep, though he seemed reticent to discuss where he had been or what he had done in the interim. Now, however, he was hungry, tired, and cold, and he needed help.

At 10:00 a.m., when the KAD office staff arrived to begin the day, Mahesh was already waiting outside the gate. He had come looking for work and shelter, and he hoped that someone here would be able to help him find either or both. This role as a landing pad for deaf migrants to the city is a familiar and fundamental part of KAD's work. Everyone involved with the organization has experience facilitating this process of social integration to some extent or another. Critically, however, this is one of the relatively few tasks deemed too important for hearing interpreters to manage on behalf of the deaf leadership. If Mahesh wanted support, he would have to wait until a deaf person came to provide it. The staff on duty did their best to assess Mahesh's more immediate needs, offered him a hot meal, and then asked him to stay until the KAD president could come. With nowhere else to go, he seemed content to do so. Mornings are typically quiet at KAD, and on days without scheduled programs it is often just the interpreters sitting by the phones, managing paperwork, and making tea until well into the afternoon. I had come in early that day to manage some paperwork myself, and Mahesh and I ended up talking for nearly three hours before someone more useful to him ultimately arrived.

Our communication was difficult but not impossible, and it got easier as time went on. I was curious about how Mahesh came to be where he sat, and Mahesh wanted to know everything I could tell him about the city. We shared, as far as I could tell, exactly no linguistic code. He had had no contact with speakers of NSL up to this point in his life, and his relationship with spoken Nepali (though significant) was mediated by perceptual acuities and forms of knowledge that I lacked. To the deaf, speech is hosted by patterns of sight and reflexes of motion that are notoriously difficult to reconstruct from the outside. The difference between a [b] and a [p], for example, is made primarily by the timing of vibrations deep in throat. Several deaf people I knew could sometimes recover the traces of this articulatory gesture by watching carefully the shape taken by a speaker's lower lip, though usually, they said, this was possible only with individuals they knew very well. Mapping speech in these terms demands staggeringly nuanced techniques of attention, as the materialities of sight and sound align in only the most scattered of ways.

This set of difficulties is the basis of the ambiguities that shroud Mahesh's name. Early in the conversation, I asked him his name, and I am certain that he understood the question. He asked me mine, in any case, and he seemed satisfied by the written, spoken, and signed representations I was able to produce for him. But Mahesh didn't read or write, and odds are that his family members didn't either. His experience of his own name, likewise, was built purely from the visual chaff of a substance privileged as sound. Mahesh knew his name as a jaw movement, one that included a bilabial closure at the beginning, a dental closure at the end, and a forward movement of the tongue blade in between.

This gesture, in a very real sense, *is* Mahesh's name, at least to the extent that his name truly is his own and not a thing lent to him by his parents and priests. This is not simply a question of modality preferences. "Mahesh" is a common name in Nepal, and its utterance produces characteristics visually similar to what Mahesh does with his jaw to name himself. But (to my untrained eye, at least) many other names do, too. His parents might just as easily have called him Manish, Ramesh, Dinesh, or any number of other possibilities that I would have been unable to distinguish reliably. This fact of irresolvability, however, is fundamentally at odds with everything that is culturally important about having a name in the first place. As a class of words, personal names are unusual for their complete lack of intensional semantics: they do not sort the world into classes of things that we might define according to a set of characteristics. It is not generally useful, for example, to talk about all the Maheshes of the world. Rather, what makes any particular Mahesh a "Mahesh" is nothing more and nothing less than the fact that other people have called him such (Quine 1960, 177). The purpose of providing a name is thus not to identify a member of a class but rather to characterize a history of reference, beginning at some critical point in the past and converging in the present on an individual. Along these very same lines, what Mahesh does with his jaw to identify himself is an echo of his name's past instances of utterance, but in this manifestation it is illegible to the hearing as such. In an ideal world, I would find a way to write Mahesh's name as it exists for him—as motion rather than as sound—but without such an architecture of conventions I am left instead guessing at what his name was for his parents.

Our talk was built from engagements with similar kinds of limits. Though he never made it explicit, Mahesh demonstrated through his actions a nuanced and complex theory of meaning, built from a lifetime of being understood without shared language as a crutch. Specifically, he knew—with deaf precision—that he would be understood only to the extent that he could render his signs in terms shaped by the aspects of our mutual past most salient to both of us. This is a significant technical challenge. Anyone can figure out, perhaps, that elephants are more notable for their long trunks than for their large feet, but it takes significantly more skill to talk about "Kathmandu," "the president of KAD," and "good places to work nearby." Thus, when I say that Mahesh managed the intelligibility of his words, I do not mean merely that he made his language understandable. Instead, his acts of meaning worked precisely to the extent that he could foreground the social histories that establish a link between words and things. He knew, specifically, that our talk depended on his ability to gauge what extent of these histories I was experiencing in context with him.

We began with a very narrow basis of mutual expectancy, built from the presences, perceptions, and sensations that we each assumed would be readily transparent to the other. As our conversation accumulated a history of shared experiences over time, however, we were increasingly able to build on what we had already established. This elaboration of our own discursive past allowed us to apply more complexly implicated deixis, more broadly mediated iconicity, and more finely tuned framings of intersubjective knowledge. I first asked Mahesh about his cooking pot:

that thing.carried.with.two.hands round.things inside you?[1]

To say this, I pointed at the pot where it sat on the floor, gripped two imaginary handles in the space in front of me that corresponded roughly to the shape, size, and placement of handles on the material pot, and oscillated the elevation of my arms a few times with a cadence indicating that it was moderately heavy. At this point, I kept my left hand gripped to the discursive pot handle, released my right hand, and arced it around to the inside of the shape. When I pulled my hand back out, my fingers were clawed in a grip around a round object the size of a potato. I rotated my hand around the discursive potato to trace its shape,

---

1. In my transcriptions here and elsewhere, I have adopted some conventions from the sign language linguistics literature. CAPITALIZED words represent standardized lexical tokens, especially those found in the official NSL dictionary. Lower case words are those I understand to have been invented creatively in real time. When a single sign requires multiple English words to represent it, these have been joined. with.periods. Question marks indicate a furrowed brow, a forwarded chin, and/or other facial features used to mark phrases as soliciting information.

then pointed at Mahesh while I pushed my chin forward in a manner familiar throughout Nepal as indicating a question. He nodded and explained:

yes stomach.pains eat-eat-eat

What I have glossed here as "stomach.pains" is a particularly important kind of sign, one that demonstrates a very visual orientation to the question of embodiment. Mahesh placed his hand over his stomach, hunched his shoulders, grimaced, and curved his back forward. This is, presumably, precisely what he did when he actually experienced the palpable and visible discomfort of hunger he is describing here. He was counting on the fact that I could imagine what he was feeling based on what he was doing because, he presumed, I had seen people do it before. Perhaps I had even experienced it myself.

I again grabbed the handles of my discursive pot, slid my left hand palm-side up underneath flat against its bottom, and touched the bent fingers of my right hand to the back of my left rapidly and repeatedly. The visuals here are particularly difficult to convey in written form, but with my sign I was trying to evoke the memory of a fire from a pressurized stove blasting against the bottom of a pot:

COOK?

I wanted to know how he cooked his food. Incidentally, this was actually the sign designated by the NSL dictionary to match the English word "cook" (figure 6), but Mahesh of course had no way to know this. Instead, I was hoping to draw his attention to something that sat under his pot, flicking with the shape and intensity of a flame from a kerosene or LPG burner. This was a bit of a gamble, however, since at this point I still had no idea where he'd come from or if he was familiar with the visuals of cooking with gas. Nevertheless, he understood, and he went on to explain:

trees.occupying.area one.tree chop-chop-chop fall

For this, he grabbed his right forearm with his left hand and rotated his right hand radially, forming a sign (coincidentally) identical to the ASL word for "tree." He reduplicated his tree a dozen or so times in the area around the front of his body, and finally stopped for a moment on one particular instance, singling out a single tree from amidst the forest. He removed his left hand and

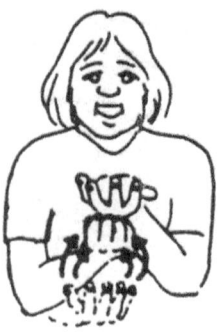

पकाउनु

Figure 6. COOK

began to chop at the base of the tree with it. After a few strikes, Mahesh's right-hand tree fell down to become horizontal. We talked for a while about how, here in the city, simply cutting down trees in forests would probably not go over well with local authorities. To do this, we established a contrast between the space immediately between us and the space eighteen inches to our side. THERE, at his village, chopping down trees was okay maybe, but HERE, in the space of Kathmandu that we now shared, these actions were blocked (the blades of two hands forming an X). He explained that he understood. He had lived at home in close proximity to a forest that was protected first by the government and later by the Maoists, so he was not naïve about the hazards of property. Here, he knew, he would have to find other ways to cook his dinner.

Each of these signs followed the trajectories described above. Some matched the forms from standard NSL that I was predisposed to, and others emerged from the idiosyncrasies of our talk. Periodically, the interpreters would jump in with questions composed in narrowly standard NSL, and at these moments Mahesh was unable to understand what was being said. Nevertheless, he recognized the existence of these conventions, and he understood their importance for both his present and his future. He frequently asked me how to say things he felt to be particularly relevant in "their sign," and moving forward he would alternate with no obvious pattern I could discern between "their" signs and "ours."

We continued like this for the entire length of our conversation. Words came to take relatively stable shape through erosions of synecdoche: pieces of more elaborate productions reduced down to simpler form but remaining referentially effective because they invoked the shared memory of a previous larger whole. The wall by the TV became a directional reference to his home to the west, for example, though we realized later that we had gotten disoriented and that the TV actually sat to the north of us. The word "tree" was reduced down to a splayed hand shaking twice along the axis of the arm. A single hand gripping a horizontal object palm up came to reference his cooking pot and, eventually, also the idea of possessions generally. These names always required more elaboration in their first invocation, but they carried forward with relatively little effort once they had been established.

Eventually, two prominent deaf signers—the president of KAD and another important member of the board—arrived to assist with the situation. Calls were made, favors were invoked, and a place was found for Mahesh. Though he was homeless and unemployed, he had the good fortune to be young, healthy, and male. Thanks to his newly found deaf peers, he now had a shared room to sleep in and a job that would pay him just enough to stay fed. By aligning pasts and futures in this way, deaf social networks and deaf languages organize a common framework of ethics. When people like Mahesh arrive in Kathmandu, the deaf community is ready to provide them with a shared past and future. This is a familiar role for KAD to play, and it demonstrates the prosthetic functions of kinship and sociality that deaf organizations often provide.

As Mahesh stepped outside to leave for the lodgings that had been arranged for him, he stopped abruptly and gathered together the attentions of everyone in the room. He had suddenly realized that all of his belongings remained in the office, and he was worried about their security. He wanted to talk about them with us, and he wanted for us to talk about them with each other. This was highly purposeful communication: Mahesh was looking to be reassured that others recognized the value he placed on his things, and he wanted to coordinate everyone's intentions in ways that would protect them. In the most tangible terms, helping Mahesh meant talking in effective ways about his cooking pot and the objects it contained. The manner in which that unfolded demonstrates the nuanced attentions to how meaning comes to be that are so often at the core of deaf language.

As would be expected, Mahesh referenced his belongings with the reduced pot-handle sign that he and I had gradually established earlier. As is perhaps *less* expected, the deaf leaders also used this local lexical anchor even after Mahesh had left the room. More specifically, they alternated freely between it and the conventional NSL lexical sign for "things" (or, at least, without any pattern intelligible to me) (figure 7). These alternations became more distinctly purposeful after Mahesh returned, however. When the deaf leaders wanted to assure him that they would figure out how to keep his belongings safe, for example, they used the indexically local pot-handle sign. When they wanted to talk privately—when, for example, they joked that nobody in the city wanted to steal a bunch of moldy potatoes—they used the distally anchored sign from the NSL dictionary. Talking to Mahesh involved a confluence of the standard forms of NSL that predate and exclude him and the highly proximal lexical anchors that he and I elaborated in the here-and-now. This lamination emerged from a complex interplay of chained back-references moving forward in time, first between Mahesh and the deaf leaders, then among the deaf leaders alone, and then again between the deaf leaders and me. Aspects of whatever shades of local signing Mahesh used at home seem to have combined with elements of the Kathmandu standard, along with countless felicitous innovations on the way. To a significant extent, what transpires here can be understood as an emerging pidgin (cf. Garrett 2008), though even that framing fails to account for the sheer speed with which these signs appear and fade. Instead, this talk about cooking pots came to depend on lineages of use and repetition that materialized the organization of our perceptual logics and extended them well beyond their original scope. These vectors of citation, often passing unseen in hearing communication, are precisely what deaf signers experience as most intelligible in the act of communication.

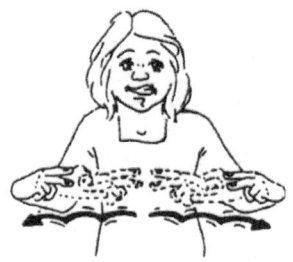

सामान/वस्तु

Figure 7. THINGS

What I mean to draw attention to here is the capacity of language to manifest in the shared perceptual space of two or more people the presence of objects with their social histories intact. Words don't mean things on their own. Though technologies like dictionaries and Necessary Words lists can erase their own conditions of possibility for experience in the here-and-now, the deaf are always keenly attentive to the history of meaning because there is so little they can take for granted about what they share linguistically with others. Moreover, because words and phrases never stand on their own without a sense of instrumental purpose, acts of speech are possible only to the extent that they congeal intentions. The deaf spend tremendous energy trying to make these intentions intelligible, disentangling the shape of signs from what they mean, why they mean it, and what these meanings reflect about other minds. Signed language, as it weaves people together in collaborative, world-facing dispositions, entangles them together in a shared world of things sensibly present.

A year later, I asked around about Mahesh, but nobody really seemed to remember him. His story is familiar enough at KAD that it had become increasingly difficult with the passage of time to single out the individual against the archetype. Deaf language in Nepal comprises a speech community with a remarkable range of participants, and these participants bring with them an expansive heterogeneity of semiotic orientations and competencies of form. These competencies—incorporating both shared lexical knowledge and intuitions of visual salience—demonstrate not signing's limits but rather its very core. I do not mean to suggest that Mahesh is in any sense exemplary as a signer, but rather these kinds of encounters between widely diverse signers are themselves exemplary of NSL. What signers know how to do—with astonishing precision—is to manage their own transparency by managing the intelligibility of meaning, manifest as a social history of names.

LANGUAGE AS A THING SEEN

Sign language is fun. That's the consensus, at least, among the hearing people I interviewed while preparing this book. It's just one of those things that everyone seems to like talking about. During the first few months of my fieldwork especially, I was overwhelmed by the number of unsolicited calls and emails I received from otherwise distant acquaintances who wanted to meet with me to talk about sign. These were not activists or anyone else with a vested interest in public understandings of the deaf. They often had no particular point to drive home, and they stood to gain nothing tangible by spending a few hours of their busy lives in this way. Nevertheless, a great many people were both gracious and persistent in their desire to share with me some specific, personal, and compelling memory about signing. This was most decidedly not the case when I asked about religious practice, movies, medicine, cooking, traditional wood-carving, leprosy, ethnonationalist politics, or cricket. Whereas those topics were often evaded as boring, controversial, or embarrassing, my questions about sign language consistently yielded both delight and hours of tape.

The stories I heard were widely diverse in politics and sophistication, but nearly all of them arrived at the same conclusion: sign language is *surprising*. Some people noted, for example, that sign language could be used to talk about an unexpectedly wide variety of things. They told me about signed versions of physics lectures curated by universities, about signed interpretations of hip hop lyrics offered on stage at concerts, about signed translations of the Ramayana and the Bible on YouTube, and about love poems, legal agreements, cooking shows, and comedy routines all done in sign. Among those who had acquired some extent of training in a sign language, everyone seemed to have strong opinions about its degree of difficulty: many noted with enthusiasm that it was unexpectedly easy to learn, and many others said that it was unexpectedly hard; exactly no one, meanwhile, described it as how they thought it would be. Further afield, one person I interviewed even went so far as to suggest that the monkeys at Swayambhunath temple seemed to be communicating with each other using something that *looked like* signing, and he wondered with obvious delight whether the deaf could maybe understand them. Beneath these various observations was a single consistent juxtaposition: sign language, marvelously, is somehow more capable than those who use it. It is a thing identified with the deaf, but it extends also through and beyond them. Frequently, these descriptions were concluded with a nod to the remarkable scope of possibility demonstrated by language generally: "*Bhāshā yastai pani hunchha, hai?*" (Language can even be like that, huh?). In the rest of this chapter, my aim is to understand these hearing expectations and to characterize the range of deaf linguistic practices that manage them.

On one Saturday morning, early in this project's fieldwork, I was sitting in the home of a midlevel official in the Ministry of Education. I was there to ask for an interview, and I had been instructed by his housekeeper to wait in a clean and brightly decorated parlor set to the side of the main house. In another chair sat a man in his early thirties. He was dressed in modest but immaculate clothing, and the oversized suitcase he carried with him suggested that he had come here straight from the bus station. As we waited together quietly over the next hour, he sifted through a small stack of documents and spoke softly to himself. He seemed to be rehearsing something, likely whatever it was he planned to say when he was finally invited into the next room. As is customary, a television was left on for our benefit, though neither of us was paying much attention to it. The chatter of sitcoms joined the din of the street immediately outside, and the space was filled with a loud white noise. The man shuffled his papers, I shuffled my feet, and both of us waited. Abruptly, a familiar chord progression escaped the television's hum to announce that the midday news broadcast would be commencing shortly on the national station. This sound is heard several times per day, but as is customary on Saturdays, today's broadcast was being given simultaneously in spoken Nepali and NSL.

When the program began, my companion abruptly stopped what he was doing to watch. His shift in bodily affect was palpable. After an hour of restless fidgeting directed at nothing in particular, he was suddenly captivated. At one point, I started to say something, but without taking his eyes off the screen he gestured for me to wait. For a full ten minutes, he sat motionless and silent. What he saw held his attention so entirely that he seemed frozen in place. When the broadcast finally ended, he turned to me with an electric grin and said, "Did you see that?!" By all indications, he was thoroughly impressed, and he seemed to think that I should be too. I asked if he had seen sign language on the news before. He explained that, yes, of course he had, but more importantly he had grown up in a village with a deaf boy roughly his age. The remarkable thing here, though, was just how different the signing on TV was from the signing he saw as a child. They were both "deaf language/talk" (*bahirako kurā*), but "this sign language was not like that sign language." The man immediately began to speculate about why:

This boy's signing was pure (*suddha*). It was always understandable. You could watch him and know what he was saying. Sometimes he would talk too fast or become too angry—it's like his body became hot—and then his talk would become unclear. But this woman [the newscaster] . . . I didn't understand a word! It was all . . . [waves his hands furiously in front of his face]. But look at her. She is presenting the news on national television. She is dressed in nice clothes and she is very pretty. She is "middle class" [in English]. The boy in the village? We were all very poor. He's probably breaking rocks for a living now. But I could always understand him. He was *sojho*.

This last word—*sojho*, generally glossed as "simple" or "straightforward"—is a complexly implicated term in Nepali. To be *sojho* is to be earnest or sincere, often to extremes. People with primary cognitive deficits are sometimes called *sojho* euphemistically, but a lack of intelligence is in no way essential to the meaning of the word. Rather, *sojho* people are inflexibly honest and often abused, but their disadvantage is more a symptom of troubled times than any personal fault of their own. In a world where things are frequently not as they seem, the *sojho* live their lives utterly without guile.

What this framing of *sojho* reflects is a distinct way of thinking about the nature of social particularity itself, one with deep consequences for the deaf. As I have argued over the past two chapters, the stigma of deafness in contemporary Nepal articulates around the premise of an inescapable transparency. Against the more general intuition that social life is built from vast, lateral entanglements of intention and context, deaf people are burdened with the expectation of being only and exactly as they appear. What the deaf supposedly lack in this regard is engagement with the patterns of opacity that accompany historically accrued regimes of knowledge and meaning, manifest in day-to-day life as webs of contextual specificity intelligible to some but not others. In its place, the deaf garner an unusual and very limited kind of agency, characterized by the near-total absence of interiority perceived within them. They are coherent as actors, perhaps, but they harbor no secrets. They are, in these terms, archetypically *sojho*. Simply by being opaque in her signing, however, the newscaster on TV served to demonstrate that there are startling exceptions to the rule. *Sojho* men who now break rocks for a living are inevitably transparent, but sophisticated women who wear good clothes and wave their hands furiously are impossible to understand. This inconsistent opacity injects signing with an ambiguity constituted against broader discourses about language and difference.

For many residents of Kathmandu, the experience of language in daily life is organized by historical dynamics of privacy and access. In a country hosting thirty million people and 122 recognized languages—with a median population of only 6,500 speakers each (M. P. Lewis, Simons, and Fennig 2013)—not understanding what other people say has always been a very familiar way of knowing them (cf. Eckert 2000). Most people speak at least one language that is understood by only a fraction of the country as a whole, and even the national language Nepali is used at home by less than half of the country. After fifty ambitious years of roads and copper wires, however, geography does not bound the flows of sociality and carve exclusions in the same ways that it once did.

Language is a major player in this new politics extracted from place (cf. Harvey 1989). The population of the Kathmandu Valley, approximately three million in 2018, is growing at a rate many times greater than that of the country as a whole. These days in Kathmandu, it seems like everybody was born someplace else. Particularly conspicuous as newcomers are job-seeking domestic migrants, civil war refugees, experts imported from overseas to drive up the country's various indicators, and a diverse range of tourists with religious, adventure-seeking, or psychedelic inclinations. Though generations of travelogues have depicted Kathmandu as the sleepy capital of a homogeneous Shangri-La, the city today is cacophonously polyglot.

Over the last two decades in particular, however, trends in domestic migration and the spread of global communication networks have stratified language competencies in distinctly generational terms. Though few people in Nepal are monolingual, the sets of languages spoken by those under thirty and by those over sixty often have little overlap. This generation gap manifests in both intimate and public domains, drawing together a tangle of local and dislocated models of the self. In recent years, for example, it has become increasingly popular among affluent urbanites to employ elderly women from remote parts of the country to act as tutors of minority languages for their young children. To the parents paying good money, the appeal of these lessons is generally driven by variously politicized tensions between national and personal identity (cf. Kunreuther 2009; Whitehead 2010). For the kids, however, the experience is usually about something very different. Many of the children I spoke with described their family's "village language" as an oppressive *secret code*, used by their parents, grandparents, and aunts and uncles to speak privately with each other in public. The point of knowing a language, as they encounter it, is often that other people don't. Language classes thus offered the children access to worlds that had previously excluded them, rendering the sometimes heavy burdens of kinship at least scrutable. In the words of one nine-year-old Limbu language tutee, fingers at his temples and eyes rolling around in playful imitation of a mystic, "I want to learn Limbu to read my mother's mind."

The parents of these children, meanwhile, often remarked on the irony of the situation: ignorance of local specificities, as much as knowledge of global trends, defines the essence and engine of cosmopolitanism. These gaps of knowledge organize encounters not only with minority languages but with spoken Nepali as well. One mother I knew, for example, complained that her thirteen-year-old son was unwilling to shop at the local market. When tasked with buying vegetables for dinner, he would instead walk twenty minutes out of his way to patronize a nearby supermarket chain. She interpreted this choice as an expression of economic aspiration, driven perhaps by his fondness for American sitcoms and a desire to participate in the kinds of consumption he witnessed therein. In these new orientations, however, she worried that he would miss out on the noise and atmosphere of the market that she loved so much as a child. She worried, specifically, that he would always lack the skills necessary to navigate these distinctly Nepali urban spaces. As it turns out, her son shared her concerns. Though he was adamant that he would never admit it to her, he acknowledged to me that he found the local bazaars disorienting. He preferred to shop at the supermarkets, he explained, not because he longed for something they offered but simply because the cash registers there used digital displays. The problem was simple: the number system in spoken Nepali is irregular all the way up to one hundred, and he sometimes had trouble remembering the word for anything much past twenty. The vegetable sellers in the local markets had apparently picked up on this fact, and they enthusiastically ridiculed him for it. In comically exaggerated rural accents, they called him *kuire* ("whitey/ foreigner," lit. "foggy"), and they asked him to bring their daughters to *Amrikā* (America). By adopting these trappings of unsophistication, they mocked the utility of his expensive English-medium education. They directed his attention to the divisions it drew between him and them, and they reminded him of just how much he still depended on them—even for something as simple as carrots.

In this broader historical context, what makes sign language so delightful is thus the possibility that it might offer an exception to the very difficult political realities of language generally. Over the last few decades especially, the stakes of linguistic difference in Nepal have taken on an uncomfortable urgency, realized primarily as friction between the country's vast ethnolinguistic diversity and its very centralized political institutions (Bandhu 1989; Sonntag 1995; Turin 2004; Giri 2011). As a consequence of these tensions, a great many people are currently either angry about language or tired of talking about it. This is especially true in the years since the fall of the monarchy and the subsequent rise of a new, ambiguously unified Nepal. Language—to the very significant extent that it is entangled by questions about self-determination and identity—has become politically dangerous. Signing, however, is different. It feels strangely accessible even to hearing people who have never learned it, and the community it organizes has no overt ambitions to kinship, ethnicity, or regional autonomy. As a consequence, what signing reveals for many is the possibility of difference without division. In the words of one enthusiastic hearing nonsigner, "Maybe there'd be less fighting in the world if everyone could talk in sign."

Though this optimism that new modalities of communication might break down arbitrary social boundaries is widespread, it rests on a profound misconception: that sign language is *universal*. When it is experienced as transparent, many hearing people assume that it extends beyond the historical limits that make Nepali, Limbu, or English available to some but not others. This expectation is overwhelmingly common in both Nepal and the West, though it articulates around some very different frameworks of intuition in each case. In the United States, anyone with even peripheral involvement with sign is familiar with how reluctant the hearing can be to grant signed languages the same possibility of variation that spoken languages have. It's something signers talk about, and perhaps every "Deaf Culture 101"-style text includes an explanation about how and why signed languages are different in different deaf communities. Critically, however, these assumptions of universality are almost always tacit; it's not something people assert as true so much as something they are surprised to learn is false. On one occasion, while talking to the director of a large voter inclusion program run by a multinational NGO, I had to explain that the interpreter he was recruiting from Thailand likely wouldn't be much help to Nepal's deaf community. After a long pause, he replied, "I guess that makes sense. But wouldn't it be better if all deaf people used the same language?"

In Nepal, by contrast, the premise of universality is generally more explicit, tied not to unscrutinized hopes for how the world might be better but instead to deep intuitions about how it already is. Specifically, when people talk about the transparency of signing, they often do so by identifying it as "*prakṛtik*." In a general sense, *prakṛti* refers to the timeless natural world and the forces within it, but critically the term does not carry with it any of the appeal to origins or authenticity that the term "natural" might in European philosophical traditions. Rather, the opposite of *prakṛtik* is not "artificial" but "intentional." *Prakṛti* is the other side of consciousness, uniting the scope of all substance independent of thought. In the course of our conversation, my waiting-room companion repeatedly called the signing he saw back in his village "*prakṛtik*," and in so doing he was identifying it as both intrinsic to and vastly larger than the boy who used it. These "natural signs" existed, he said, before the various races (*jāt*) of people scattered and evolved. They are profoundly human in character, but critically they have no history. They present instead the possibility of language without the compromising entanglements of agency or design.

For the deaf, these ascriptions to the preconscious are a very mixed blessing. Though the deaf are very eager to share their love of signing with absolutely anyone, the hearing's enthusiasm for sign is made complicated by the some-times very strange things that they want it to be. Early in my fieldwork, for example, I was puzzled by how frequently I heard signing described as a "*dhar-mic* language," a phrase more typically reserved for Sanskrit, Pali, Tibetan, and other liturgical languages. I interpreted this attribution initially as a gesture of generosity, meant as a euphemistic expression for the low status generally ac-corded the deaf. A more nuanced understanding, however, can be found in the particulars of *dharmic* existence in South Asia and how the meaning invoked by the word is different from its sometimes-translation "religion."

To call *dharma* a moral or ethical law (as is often done) will bring us to the right ballpark of meaning while simultaneously missing the point entirely. *Dharma* is an account not of how things ought be but rather of how they already are. It is the basic underlying organizational coherence of the universe, and all one can do is to act in harmony or disharmony with it. Certainly nonviolence and food taboos are questions of *dharma*, but—equally—so is the manner in which a stone rolls down a hill. This experience of essential and unshakable presence is precisely what comes to be at stake in claims about the "natural" basis of signing. According to this reckoning, deaf communicative modes exist in a way basic to the world itself, unmodified and unmotivated by anything less comprehensive than the universe in its entirety. The fact that sign language *works* does not serve to prove any broader historical engagement by deaf com-munities. Rather, it only goes to show that linguistic transparency is itself the natural order of things in the absence of social history. Opacity is the distortion.

Just as so-called "wolf children" provided Enlightenment thinkers with an opportunity to gaze upon human nature in its (ostensibly) barest form (Itard 1842), signing in Nepal is made to stand as a demonstration of language free from everything else. The idea here is that opacity is not inevitable but rather an *effect* of accumulated social particularity, a thing supposedly lacked by the boy in my waiting-room companion's village but held in excess by the woman newscaster. The opacity of television signing thus comes about as a distortion of language's otherwise basic shape, driven not by the nature of signs but rather by signers entangled in contextually distinct regimes of historical contingency.[2]

---

2.   Joel Robbins (2001) has argued that, in particular, ritual language (such as the self-consciously performative dimensions of television speech) reveals the extent

In these terms, when my companion experienced the signing newscaster as opaque, what he was experiencing was his own sense that she was like himself. She was "middle class," just like him, and she participated in the architectures of gender, fashion, and public voice that oriented him as well. It was this basis of commensuration through recognizable forms of difference that, ironically, explained why she was impossible to understand. As a consequence, her opacity served to prove the complexity of her interior self. The boy back in the village, meanwhile, could always be understood, but only because he was so unlike other people. He was *sojho*, and his way of talking was *prakṛtik*. Like Arjun before him, he was too easily known to demand recognition as a mind. The juxtaposition of these very different signers aligned to demonstrate for my companion an unexpected possibility: *signing is as it is because signers are as they are*. It's not that the deaf *lack* mind, exactly, but rather that their nonopacity demonstrates a mind unentangled by context and history. When signing is done by someone more socially entangled such as this newscaster, however, it becomes opaque as well.

To the deaf, these expectations are tremendously frustrating. Indeed, the most common complaint I heard from the deaf about hearing attempts at signing is just how bad they are at it. Sometimes, when the hearing want to communicate something but don't know how, they will even *make up* new signs on the spot. These are not guesses from context nor even appeals to pantomime. Instead, with remarkable frequency, the hearing will assemble actual gibberish and hope that it might be understood. These "fake signs" even follow a consistent formal pattern. On the many occasions that I saw them or heard them described, they would usually be made with a single dominant hand, resting palm out just below neck level. With a rigidly featureless facial expression, the fake signer then flicks his or her wrist with a spastic wiggle of fingers intended to mean . . . something. In these moments, the hearing position themselves very explicitly within their own ideologies of sign's inherent transparency: simply by moving one's hands and thinking about an answer, communication should flow.

It is no surprise perhaps that the deaf experience their part in these encounters very differently. Though hearing people were often eager to share with me their recollections of just how easy it can be to communicate with the deaf, the

---

to which local intuitions about denotation shape expectations of language efficacy. Likewise, Miyako Inoue's work on the tacit histories that emerge from women's speech practices strongly suggests that the opposition between village sign and television sign might articulate a kind of "natural history" of different kinds of deaf people (Inoue 2004).

deaf themselves more frequently described the demands of being transparent to the hearing as exhausting. Because the hearing don't sign, the deaf must create for them signs that will be transparent from the ground up with every new instance of encounter. This requires careful estimations about what is and isn't salient to them in a given context, and mobilizing these intuitions into actual linguistic form requires immense creativity. It requires knowing, for example, that water and tea are usually best distinguished not with reference to their color or temperature but rather by the shape of the vessel most characteristically used to serve them. It requires knowing that mobile phones are still imagined as things you hold against your head, even though voice-based calling has long been displaced by texting and social media as their primary mode of use. It requires knowing that people visualize bread as something eaten with two hands, that they recognize women primarily by their nose piercings, and that they will usually understand barking to indicate a dog—if it is done with a proper underbite. What signing with the hearing requires, in short, is a nuanced understanding of what they perceive about the world.

What drives the transparency of signing, thus, is not an unfettered translation of the world into symbols but rather an elaborate set of deaf intelligibility practices, constituted through careful attention to hearing habits of perception and notice. This includes nuanced estimations of hearing minds and calculations about what will or will not be obvious to the hearing in a given context (cf. Husserl 1960, especially Meditation V). In other words, however capably the deaf and the hearing might sometimes communicate,[3] what is most important is just how differently each perceive their own part in the communication. In the course of the fieldwork for this book, I watched this asymmetry unfold countless times. That deaf boy back in the village no doubt *seemed* transparent to those around him, but this fact of seeming was possible only because the *actual* burden of transparency fell solely upon him. When his signing was intuitive, it was intuitive because he had tailored it—carefully and self-consciously—to the very local context of experience he shared with those around him. He knew what they would understand, and he knew what things were most visually present to them in the world around them. His transparency was built through the mobilization of these vast storehouses of contextual knowledge, entangling the

---

3.   There is a growing body of literature on this topic of deaf–hearing interactions in language (cf. Morford and Goldin-Meadow 1997; Coppola 2002; Morford 2002; Torigoe and Takei 2002).

formal properties of his signs with shared orientations around a much broader social memory. These histories of evaluation and intention are what constitute the efficacy of deaf talk, and yet more often than not they go completely unnoticed by the hearing. In these moments, deaf language is least intelligible precisely when it is most easily understood.

Our newscaster, in contrast, faces no such burden of anticipating a particular other in a particular time and place. To the contrary, TV is famous for its power to address both everyone and no one at once, constituting a public without engaging anyone specifically. In the case of bilingual NSL broadcasts, these aesthetics of depersonalized sociality serve to anonymize not only the audience but the speaker as well. Though our newscaster—"dressed in nice clothes" and "very pretty"—faced directly into the camera as she signed, her visual engagement was supplanted by a series of Nepali-language voiceovers. These voiceovers alternated at each segment break between male and female, stripping from them even the perceptual possibility that they might belong to her or to any other particular individual. Though the act of signing was fixed to a single visible body, the substance of meaning accessible to the hearing was displaced to voices most notable for *lacking* any fixed location or identity.

Paradoxically, it is this same boundless generality that made the signing on television so opaque to the man I watched with. As anonymous language, it was aligned not to a particular set of social coordinates but rather to a set of conventions—grammar, vocabulary, genre—that constitute language *outside* of a specific instance of use. What village signing and signing on television represent are thus antipodes of social context. They organize contrastive modalities of signing because they emerge from radically different environments of shared knowledge and experience. They create reference to things in the world, respectively, through knowledge of the visual intuitions maintained by others or through knowledge of historical conventions. Signers mobilize these differences strategically for a variety of communicative and other social ends.

Though my waiting-room companion perceived in his experience of sign a basic and insurmountable difference between neighborhood boys and TV presenters, the difference he perceived was not actually about *them* but rather overwhelmingly a displacement of their relationship with *him*. They engaged him, differently, as either a particular person in a particular time and place or as an anonymous member of a television public. His encounters with transparency and opacity were thus shaped by very different histories of linguistic practice that he didn't even notice as there. This nonperception of contingency is what allows the hearing to understand signing as "natural," but—ironically—the natural here is made possible by the sheer vastness of signing's entanglement by social context. However much the hearing might experience deaf language as intrinsically transparent, transparency is itself never passive or accidental (cf. Kendon 1980; Taub 2001). Instead, being transparent takes work.

For the deaf, signing always comes with a choice. The deaf can accommodate the hearing by crafting their signs in ways that maximize their accessibility to nonsigners, but in so doing they serve to affirm every naturalistic assumption held by the hearing about deaf people and their ostensible lack of subjective interiority. Alternately, they can orient their signs around the conventions of grammar and vocabulary particular to the deaf community in Kathmandu, but these alignments then exclude the hearing from the most useful parts of communication. When the hearing *see* language, what they perceive are the complex and shifting presences that constitute signs in a time and place. What they consistently fail to see, however, are the intentions, motivations, and vectors of citation that make these elaborations possible. As distinct aspects that unify language, the meaning of signs and the social history of signing are both necessary conditions in all moments of engagement between the deaf and the hearing. Each comes to be present in hearing worlds, however, only at the expense of the other. At any given moment, either can be seen, but both cannot.

THE INTELLIGIBILITY OF WORDS

The *Nepali Sign Language Dictionary* is a remarkable achievement. Since its publication in 2004, thousands of copies have circulated both within Nepal and internationally. The dictionary contains 2,202 words, gathered by a deaf task force over more than a decade in consultation with hundreds of signers from across the country. As an explicit foundation for competency in NSL, the dictionary has become an important tool for both teaching and standardizing the language. As a document legitimizing the place of sign language in education, media, and governance, it has made possible a new era of institutional sanction for deaf Nepal.

Printed on coarse A4 paper and bound with staples inside a brightly designed clipart cover (figure 8), the dictionary contains 159 pages divided into 33 thematic chapters. Each page is subdivided with thick black lines into 16 panels in a 4 × 4 grid. Within each of these boxes is a single hand-drawn illustration accompanied by glosses in both English and written Nepali. Though these images are highly unified in style and organization, there is conspicuously no attempt to decompose them into a fixed inventory of recombinable sublexical segments. The dictionary does not, in other words, build its vocabulary from anything equivalent to an alphabet or a phonemic inventory. Furthermore, as Erika Hoffmann-Dilloway (2008) has argued, the NSL dictionary establishes a firmly lexicalist understanding of language. It describes a strictly dyadic correspondence between signs and meanings, with no further question of building up to syntax or breaking down to morphology. Rather, each picture depicts a complete human body (alternately male and female) frozen in the act of producing a complete word, with only minimal explicit cues about which parts of the picture are meant to be understood as contrastively relevant. These illustrations are the only exponents of NSL's articulatory form, and yet they remain holistic and already composed in their presentation. The NSL dictionary is, in short, a dictionary of pictures.

Dictionaries of spoken languages, meanwhile, must necessarily be organized in very different terms. Speech's acoustic signals are at inherent odds with the blank spaces of paper, and as a consequence the visual representation of spoken words requires elaborate technologies of writing to work. Though there are many proposed transcription inventories for signed languages (Stokoe, Casterline, and Croneberg 1976; Sutton 1995), none has gained much traction in Nepal or elsewhere.[4] Instead, across cultures and contexts, people seem to prefer to represent signs pictorially. As a consequence of these choices, what the dictionary most directly provides is an experience of equivalence between words and bodies, bridging the perceptual differences of speech and sign in unexpected ways (cf. Goodwin 1994).

Owing in part to these technical configurations, the dictionary has come to constitute a centrally important site of interaction between the deaf and the hearing. More than any other public intervention perhaps, this simple folio of stapled pages has transformed how hearing family members think about and participate in the communicative practices of their deaf kin. When signers leave the Kathmandu Valley to visit relatives for the Dashain holidays, for example, they often bring with them several copies of the book "just to leave around." This manner of intentional scattering accounts for the bulk of the NSL dictionary's circulation.

---

4.   See Rosenthal (2009) for a broader discussion of sign language transcription.

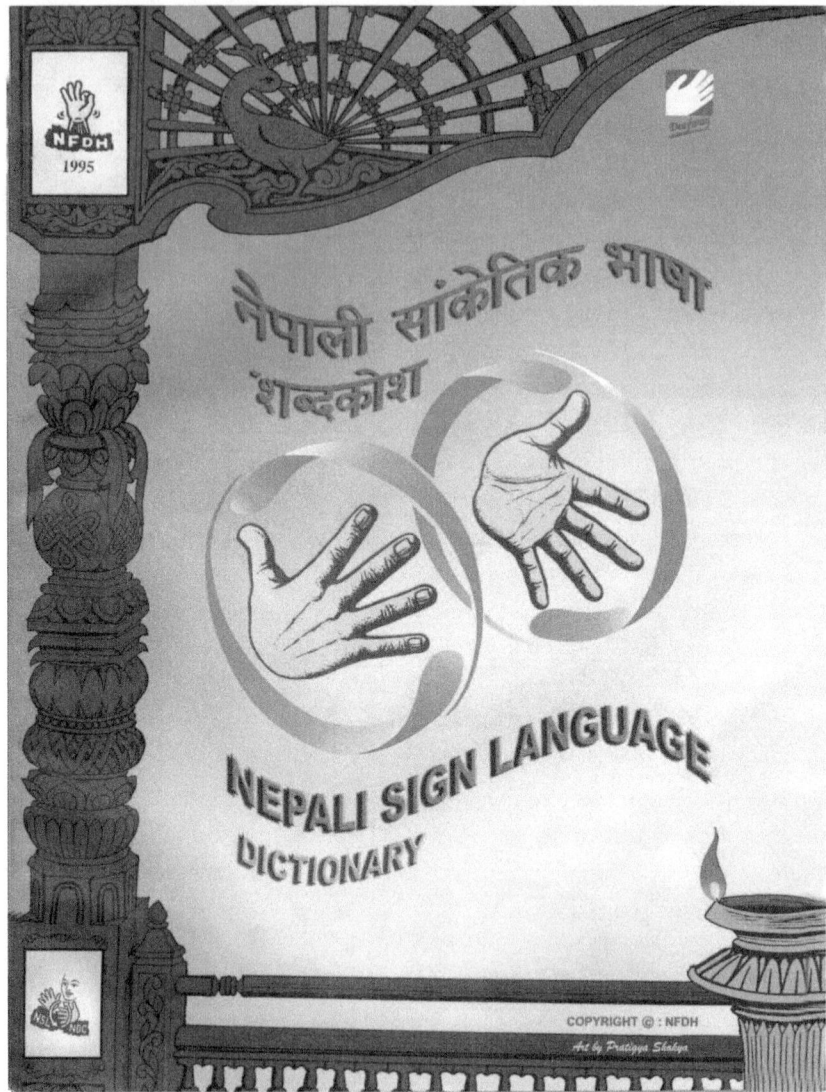

Figure 8. Cover of the *Nepali Sign Language Dictionary*

Though the dictionary is organized as a reference volume, hearing people who stumble upon it don't generally consult it as such. They don't, for example, typically search through its pages to find translations of specific words they need. Instead, in my experience at least, they *read* it. They go through its pages carefully and one at a time, most often in groups of three or four. This is no mere passive study, however. When presented with an alignment of written and drawn words, hearing people invariably start to *sign*. They make themselves *look like* the signers on the page, translating the positions and movements depicted in the dictionary onto their own bodies, and they begin speculating with obvious pleasure about *why* particular sign-shapes correspond to particular meanings. Though these attempts to explain the shapes of signs inevitably serve to reinforce the hearing belief that signing is *natural*, the tangible permanence that the book offers also gives NSL a very explicit institutional frame. It serves not only to bootstrap progressively more complicated communicative relationships between the deaf and the hearing but also to demonstrate the more technical fact that NSL is the kind of thing to require an architecture of conventions in the first place. The decision to include English glosses was a stroke of genius as well, or at the very least a fortunate accident. Though the hearing often experience signing as too inevitably transparent to constitute *language* in any conventional sense, they are frequently confronted with the opacity of English as a dimension of prestige and power. On numerous occasions, I saw hearing people use the NSL dictionary not to learn NSL but rather to study English, bypassing the stated purpose of the book while simultaneously populating the alignment of local and global languages with imagery of signers.

One thing the hearing tend not to notice when browsing, however, is the dictionary's very unusual distribution of lexical items. Among its 2,202 words, nearly ten percent are designated under the heading "Signs on the subject of organizations and offices," and another five percent fall under the categories "Constitution and government administration signs," "Signs related to sewing," and "Signs related to domestic electrical wiring." A further eight percent are the names of foods. The dictionary includes twenty-seven signs for different kinds of birds, and yet it has remarkably few signs to describe the spatial properties of material objects or the sequencing of events. There is a sign for PENGUIN, for example, but nothing glossed as "away" or "across." There is a sign meaning DEPUTY_SECRETARY, but nothing like "while," "during," or anything else that might describe one happening interrupted by another. These gaps are striking, but nevertheless I do not wish to suggest that the contents of the dictionary are somehow incomplete or skewed. Certainly, the extent of interest paid to bureaucratic matters, democratic governance, and vocational training reveals something about the circumstances of the dictionary's creation, but on the whole I believe it is accurate to say that it provides a reasonably balanced representation of NSL's standard vocabulary. Furthermore, though its collection of words is quite small as far as dictionaries go (especially considering how many of them are nouns restricted to highly specialized contextual applications), fluent signers nevertheless have a remarkably difficult time coming up with examples of words that are *missing*.

This dearth of words becomes especially conspicuous when we step outside the circles most directly involved in the dictionary's creation. As a demographic fact, the speech communities that constitute deaf Kathmandu are complexly nested. Someone like Mahesh, with no history of sustained interaction with other deaf people before his arrival in Kathmandu, represents one extreme. The typical president of KAD, meanwhile, by virtue of spending all of every work day interacting with those responsible for fixing the dictionary's content, represents another. These two poles stand sometimes in tension with each other, but the vast majority of deaf Kathmandu occupies a more flexible position in the middle. They sign fluently and effectively, but they do so with little reference to the dictionary or its contents. In ad hoc experiments I conducted with this nonstandard mainstream, for example, my participants were able to identify roughly only a quarter of the signs in the NSL dictionary when shown them in isolation. Though these unrecognized words included technical concepts like VICE_PRESIDENT, VOLUNTEER, and PADLOCK, they also included more seemingly basic terms like FAMILY, BLUE, and RICE. By any test of vocabulary, it is extremely difficult to justify the notion that these signers know NSL. Yet, by watching them sign effectively with a diverse range of others at events archetypical of deaf sociality in contemporary Kathmandu, it is equally difficult to justify the notion that they don't.

To be clear, this is not simply a question of dialect; there is no *other* set of signs that would have worked better for the purposes of this kind of elicitation. Rather, if we wish to identify NSL as the language spoken by the deaf community in its most frequent and familiar frames of interaction, we must face the paradox that its most typical speakers somehow know the language fluently with surprisingly little emphasis on what we would call vocabulary. It is empirically indisputable that nonstandard signers talk effectively with their more standard-oriented peers, but it is much more difficult to nail down what exactly it is that these two groups share in conventional linguistic terms. This question of shared knowledge runs through every register and every regional form of NSL. It foregrounds the problem of speaker competency because it makes the *content* of NSL unexpectedly hard to find.

To illustrate the descriptive problems at stake here, it is perhaps easiest to draw on an example: in the NSL dictionary, there is a sign glossed as HEAVY (figure 9). When I produced the sign for deaf activists, they told me that it meant precisely that: "heavy." When I asked them to talk about *heavy things*, however, they only very occasionally used this lexical convention to achieve their ends. More often, they chose to manifest the presence of "heaviness" in their fluent signing by relating *themselves* to the phenomenologically organized, real-world properties of the things they wanted to characterize as such. To reference a heavy backpack, for example, they did the same thing they did to reference an ordinary backpack, but they did it . . . heavier. Specifically, a "heavy backpack" is made "heavy" by the extent to which it causes a signer to bend under its weight or, alternately, to adopt a fatigued look on his or her face. The distinction being made here is built from an intuition of the effects heavy backpacks have on a person's shoulders, but it might also be achieved by any other number of things: a resulting back pain, the lumbering gait characteristic of those who have to carry heavy things while walking, or the fact that a heavy backpack must be lifted with two hands instead of just one. In all instances, a "heavy backpack" is "heavy" because it looks like what carrying a heavy backpack *feels like*. Notably, this is different from what carrying a heavy ball or heavy chair looks like. A ball is not "heavy" in the way that a backpack is "heavy," and neither is it "heavy" in the way that an elephant, a car, or a pen is (Bauman 2003; Perniss 2007; Quinto-Pozos 2007).

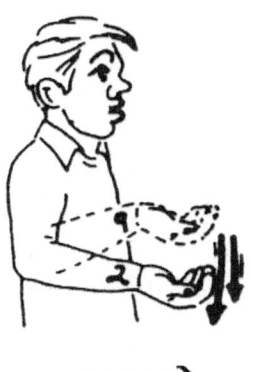

गह्ङ्गो

Figure 9. HEAVY

In this regard, to suggest that "heaviness" should obtain by virtue of a distinct and abstracted lexical item, as dictionaries tend to do, goes against the grain of NSL's very logic of organization. "Heavy" exists for the deaf not chiefly as a conventional word-form but instead as something embodied, inherently contextual, and always local. It is often not possible to distill the weight of heavy things to a corresponding sign-dyadic word because, fundamentally, the property itself resists objectification. Instead, signers communicate the fact of heaviness not through a conventional knowledge of correspondence between words and things but rather through a shared intuition about the physical world and the bodies that inhabit it. Why relegate "heavy" to an arbitrary *word* when everybody already knows what it *feels* like to manage a world of heavy things?

This attention to the problem of shared experience permeates through every dimension of linguistic function available to deaf signers in Nepal, and it leaves the parts that can be usefully isolated from context remarkably thin. This question of abstraction and separation is necessarily technical (Graif 2013), but suffice it to say that the kinds of operations that give form to "heaviness" illustrated above extend to all aspects of NSL grammar. A car might be made heavy by virtue of strained horizontal pushing, because that is how the heaviness of cars is experienced. At the same time, a frigid night is "very cold" in the sense that it modifies an underlying lexical term COLD, but the "very" here is never the same "very" that makes a furious man "very angry." Nor, however, is it productive to treat all these various degrees of cold and various degrees of anger as all independent lexical items—synonym clusters, as it were—since signers and seers can adapt between them creatively in real time. In this way, perhaps every verb of movement, every adverb of manner, every adjective of degree, every noun with visual characteristics, and every evidential or evaluative construction (not to mention anything else that can be analogized as one or more of these things) can be referenced by inhabiting the phenomenologically salient properties of the thing as it exists for oneself and for others. In Nepal, signers are always aware that they sign for *other people*, and NSL is a language that *means* things by sharing the experience of inhabiting them.

To be clear, I am not suggesting that NSL occupies a wider spectrum on an ostensible language–gesture continuum. To the contrary, I am arguing that attempts to make a distinction between NSL's formal structure and deaf Nepal's culturally anchored regimes of experience and perception are particularly fruitless. What I think these circumstances demonstrate instead—and what I think is much more broadly relevant for an ethnographic theory of language—is the remarkably peripheral role that fixed words play in NSL competency and NSL use (cf. Taub 2001; Aronoff, Meir, and Sandler 2005; Rosenstock 2008). This is as true for standard-register speakers as it is for nonstandard. Though the deaf activists involved in the creation of NSL's dictionary are generally *able* to mobilize the kinds of conventional lexical correspondences illustrated in it, in actual practice they only sometimes *do*. At least as often, they make their signs intelligible on the basis of the same kinds of productive sensory logics that nonstandard signers use. It is this shared orientation to language as a contextually elaborated thing that allows signers of widely diverse backgrounds in Kathmandu to communicate effectively with each other. Across the broad scope of NSL's practices, lexical conventions are no doubt an effective way of referring to things, but they remain only one among many. At all other moments, signers are doing something that we do not at present have adequate linguistic models to describe. What signers *know* beyond words—and what they *must* know to be fluent signers—is something else entirely.

From an analytic standpoint, there are only a few ways out of this dilemma. We could, for example, argue that this way of speaking NSL characterized by standard and nonstandard signers is not in fact actually language at all but rather something else, something gestural perhaps (see Klima and Bellugi 1979). This is not completely unreasonable, and for the purposes of analysis we can define language however narrowly we choose to justify this distinction. Nevertheless, there is something deeply unsatisfying about solving a descriptive problem simply by defining it away. At a level of basic observation, what signers do both looks like and acts like language in every sense of the term important to both Americans and Nepalis alike. It does everything language does, it gives its users the capacity to say whatever they feel motivated to say, and they show no overt interest in replacing it with anything else. The reality is far more interesting and far more challenging to represent: to speak NSL properly—even and especially in the most narrowly denotative terms—one must know what it feels like to carry a variety of heavy things.

It is these dimensions of experience that make the NSL dictionary such a strange fit with the linguistic competencies of deaf Kathmandu. The dictionary, very simply, is a dictionary of *what*. It lists in tabular form the relationships of correspondence that situate words and meanings together. The deaf, however, are by necessity less interested in facts of *what* than in logics of *how*. They must orient around these dimensions because they can take so little for granted about what they share linguistically with others. Consequently, when the deaf see language—whether with the hearing or with each other—what they see is not bare correspondences of lexical form but rather a historically anchored basis of motivation and efficacy. They see, specifically, the social processes by which words and signs come to correspond to each other amidst their own vast and shifting scopes of shared memory. The question of *how* words become intelligible is not incidental knowledge but rather fundamental to fluency in modern NSL. It is the thing that deaf people experience as most consequentially present in language's formal shape, even as it remains unseen by the hearing.

I do not mean to suggest that the NSL dictionary is naïve or misguided in its focus on lexical forms, however. To the contrary, by understanding deaf ways of engaging words as social facts, we shed new light on the dictionary's very technically oriented stock of vocabulary. After all, technical nouns are precisely the class of terms that most strongly benefit from fixed form, as it is these words that are most difficult to unfold in real-time discourse from low-level bases of mutually aligned perception. By itself, there is nothing unusual about recognizing this role for context, and this same guiding intuition shapes the efficacy of proper names in spoken languages as well (Kripke 1980). A statement about Helen Keller, for example, will invariably resolve for a wider range of people than will one about Raghav Bir Joshi, and the name Claude Lévi-Strauss can be used with impunity at an anthropology conference but only with thick contextualization at a children's birthday party. Speaking *any* language effectively requires the ability to manage these uneven landscapes of meaning and transparency, but what is remarkable about speakers of NSL is that they can extend these principles across the long tail of vocabulary until language approaches its vanishing point. They can use their language effectively with those among whom they share a comprehensive inventory of conventional words, but they can also use it to communicate with those who have never before encountered sign. All deaf people in Nepal by necessity experience language as a thing constituted by this diversity of engagements, and most of their time is spent not at either extreme but rather somewhere in the middle. In these moments of translation, we might see the NSL dictionary most clearly as a dictionary of *names*. Mahesh is "Mahesh" because other people have called him such, and HEAVY is a name for heaviness among the members of the deaf community who remember using it together. This is, however, only part of the story. When names so often cannot be counted on to make acts of reference intelligible, signers turn to something else instead.

In all of this, I am not simply arguing that language is more than code. That point has by now been so clearly demonstrated (see, e.g., Grice 1969) that to belabor it here would be tedious. Rather, I am suggesting that—even and especially as code—NSL must be understood as a system organized around the management of what is and isn't *intelligible* to others about the presence of words. Namely, words are not merely a matter of *what*, and hearing proclivities to experience them as such cannot but mythologize the language as a voice from nowhere—like so many TV newscasters speaking to an audience they cannot see. These hearing habits, acquired over a lifetime, render invisible everything that signers actually experience as most consequentially real about NSL. When language refers, it floods experience with *presences*, and it propels these *presences*, as if they were cannonballs, from one person to another. Names are useful to this end because they provide speakers of a language with an epistemologically normative way to collaborate in managing the world of things that are mutually apparent. Without these norms to always fall back on, however, the deaf must instead construct their signs from a far more sophisticated set of attentions.

CHAPTER 4

Seeing politics

These people filling the market, grab them by the eye!
Provoke them and slap them with the bam bam of God's song!
Here at this intersection, on the canvas reversed, on the field of war, in life
Stopping the sun for a moment

           – Bairāgī Kāinlā, "People Filling the Market"

INTELLIGIBILITY PLAY

According to Shyam Thapa (not his real name), it takes big eggs to work in the village. Shyam, a recent graduate of the Naxal School for the Deaf, is well known for his sometimes crude but always creative wordplay. "Eggs" here is an obvious metaphor for testicles, though, given the iconic character of the sign (wobbly round object), it is not clear that any detour away from the literal is even necessary. Then again, we were talking about the steely determination of a particular woman we both knew, so perhaps precise terminology was never really at stake here in any case. This woman, whom I'll call Rina Ghale, was about to return from several months of teaching NSL outside the Kathmandu Valley, and Shyam and I were talking—in his comfortable house, drinking cold

Orange Fanta, and watching soccer on TV—about why most deaf people are so reluctant to work in rural areas.

The problem of "centralization" is widely acknowledged in moments of self-reflection across all sectors of public service in Nepal (Lawoti 2005; Gellner 2007), but the apprehensions that deaf people bring to the issue extend well beyond those held by the typical development industry bureaucrat. Though there is near-total agreement among deaf activists that spreading NSL to the countryside is the most urgent task facing the deaf political movement, volunteering to do this work remains an act of remarkable self-sacrifice. Even and especially among the great many signers who grew up in rural areas, it can be very hard to give up the amenities, relationships, and opportunities of deaf Kathmandu. This is not, in other words, just a question of urban habits and creature comforts; there is far more to miss in the countryside than Fanta and broadcast sports.

The simple reality is that being deaf outside of Nepal's few major cities can be a miserable experience, filled with indignity and isolation. Those who have escaped these circumstances are understandably reluctant to choose to return to them. As I was sometimes told and very frequently saw myself, the hearing can be decidedly unpleasant—patronizing at best and vicious at worst—to the deaf people they encounter (Prasad 2003). Even those who mean well can be exhausting, as their deep naïveté about deaf lives builds a world of empty spaces that must be filled by activists with laborious explanations about even the most basic and obvious things. As one sign language teacher related to me, "When I go out to the village, I am working all the time. Every moment. In every tiny little thing I do, everyone watches me, saying to each other things like, 'Oh look, he likes to eat chicken. I wonder why?'" This pattern of hearing behavior is underwritten by a powerful and pervasive intuition that the deaf lack any kind of substantial interiority. The hearing project remarkably little content into the empty spaces of the deaf left by everything that cannot be seen directly. Unlike everyone else, the deaf are expected to be only and exactly as they appear, and this tacit anticipation of near-total absence within them often causes the revelation of even simple social facts to come as a surprise. It's hard to imagine hearing people asking each other *why* they enjoy chicken, and yet in encounters with the deaf even this dullest of particularities seems to justify collaborative public notice. For many deaf professionals, these assumptions of emptiness loom as a reminder of harder times, and they compromise the technically demanding work that they are called to do in rural areas. In the economy of authority that organizes Nepal's politics of development (Justice 1989; Shrestha 1997; Hindman 2009), deaf experts are plagued by the perceived impossibility of deaf expertise.

The sad and difficult reality (sometimes acknowledged and sometimes denied by activists) is that linguistic isolation leaves many deaf individuals with exactly the kinds of deficits that the hearing world expects them all to have. Against these circumstances, it is unsurprising that activists have framed their project primarily around the problem of language. This is a strategic and aesthetic decision simultaneously: if there is a single principle that unifies deaf activists in Nepal, it is sign language. They like it. They want all deaf people to know it, and they want some hearing people to know it too. As far as an explicit content goes, the value of signing is probably the only uncontested tenet of deaf politics.[1] And, to these ends, all the hard work is paying off. Despite having little institutional sanction in the hearing worlds of governance and power, the deaf have been remarkably effective in promoting their language: every year in Nepal, the number of signers grows.

To expand the reach of sign language, deaf activists travel around Nepal offering six-week to four-month courses in NSL to deaf people and their families. Over the last few decades, the structure, extent, and framing of these missions have shifted significantly with funding cycles and political priorities, but the work itself has consistently articulated around what Bateson (1972) called a double-bind: when deaf teachers arrive in rural towns, they must be both deaf enough to claim access to those they seek to teach and yet undeaf enough to appear capable of doing so. They must, in other words, establish both their equivalence to and their separation from the indigenous deaf populations they encounter. Critically, they must do all of this in sign language.

In the course of my fieldwork, I accompanied several of these expeditions outside of the Kathmandu Valley, and I visited several more that were already in progress. The work involved is undeniably arduous. After a period of training, deaf teachers set off to their assigned regions with only what they can carry to last them through the duration of their mission. They stay in boarding houses or rented rooms, and they conduct daily classes with whomever they can persuade to show up. Ideally, they maintain separate classes for the deaf and for their hearing family members, though in practice it is generally quite

---

1. In this regard I follow Green (2014), who writes persuasively that the entire scope of communicative function is framed in deaf Nepal as an ethical problem.

difficult to keep nondeaf participants motivated to attend regularly once the novelty of the program has worn off. Particularly over longer course periods, scheduled classes generally erode into private tutorials, compelling the visiting teachers to spend large parts of their day traveling from house to house visiting families with deaf members. Though the program administrators back in the city sometimes lamented this breakdown of routine, veteran teachers recognized some benefits too. It is nice to have a class, but it is often even more valuable to have intimate access to the home lives of students. There, activists can function as social workers and role models as much as teachers. A significant part of the transformative effect these programs have, I believe, is a result simply of the visible presence of an educated and articulate deaf person in town. The fact of a deaf teacher making rounds every day serves this end splendidly.

One spring shortly before the start of the monsoon, I traveled to Rasuwa District with a deaf sign language teacher in his mid-twenties I'll call Niraj. He was accompanied by Rina (the young deaf woman mentioned at the beginning of this chapter) and a hearing interpreter the two had retained for the trip. After traveling four hours by bus and another four hours on foot, we stopped for lunch a short distance from the town square where Niraj would work for the coming several months. Though the food would have been better an hour earlier along the road, the timing and position of our stop here were important. While Rina and I ate, Niraj instructed the interpreter to go on ahead. She was to find the chairman of the local Village Development Committee (VDC) and to seek his permission to operate in his town. In all reality, his blessing was probably not really necessary. For better and for worse, the stakes of deaf activism to nondeaf politics are generally low enough to draw very little attention (cf. Hankins 2009). Nevertheless, Niraj hoped the chairman would offer to organize a small gathering that evening in the town square. Sure enough, when the interpreter returned, she informed us that he had granted us his full endorsement and that he had called a town meeting so he could introduce us.

It was early evening when we finally arrived to a crowd of roughly sixty people, assembled in the dusty open space next to the town's most prominent *pipal* tree. This crowd included, I would later learn, five deaf people standing with their families, all of whom Niraj hoped would learn NSL under his tutelage. Before we arrived, Niraj had instructed me to join the audience. There, I was to respond politely to anyone who addressed me, but I should not seek out conversation. He and Rina, meanwhile, stood next to the VDC chairman without talking, watching as the crowd first gathered and then became increasingly rest-less as time drew on.

Niraj wore grey slacks and a clean but modest dress shirt. As fashion choices, these clothes seemed a nod to what Mark Liechty (2003) has called an aesthetic of middleness—neither Asian nor European and neither fashionable nor utili-tarian. This style of dress offered Niraj a displacement to nowhere, a panglobal imagery that identifies with no place in particular and thus here as much as anywhere else. Rina, on the other hand, was styled in the bright colors, intricate embroidery, and contrastively arranged tight and draping lines exemplary of Kathmandu's then latest kurta suruwal[2] fashion. Dressing this way was a strong and burdensome choice. These clothes were completely inappropriate for walk-ing in the hills, and Rina complained to us about their bulk for the entire dura-tion of the trip. Even in Kathmandu, she was not used to wearing quite so much fabric. As if to underscore her orientations to kinds of identity explicitly based elsewhere, Rina furthermore held her cell phone continually in her left hand and would occasionally manipulate its controls, this despite the fact that cellular coverage had not yet reached this part of the country. She was physically here, but her mode of comportment and self-presentation were organized entirely by connections to other places. The villagers could see the presence of these connections, but all particulars remained hidden by geographies and screens, untraceable and inscrutable for content. Niraj meanwhile just stood, rocking on his heels and watching the crowd. He kept his hands in his pockets except to occasionally check his watch.

After a delay that might have been calculated to sit just on the safe side of rudeness, Niraj and Rina stepped forward to occupy a more conspicuous position in the space. Then, Rina nodded to the interpreter, who informed the crowd that the program would begin after just five more minutes. This further wait was ostensibly designed to give any stragglers a chance to join the audience, though enough time had passed already that it was hard to imagine that anyone intending to come might realistically still be on his or her way. At that moment, however, Rina and Niraj broke the rhythms of waiting by doing something very unexpected: they began to talk to each other in sign language. The effect was an implosive silence from the audience, sudden and complete. Though most people

---

2. A style of clothing consisting of pants and a short frock, popular among young urban women as an alternative to the lunghi skirts popular in the hills and the more formal saḍi identified with India.

present had seen and even used "home signs"[3] to communicate with their deaf
kin and neighbors, I suspect that few had ever seen two deaf people—let alone
two well-dressed deaf people ascended from the city—communicating in sign
with each other. The five deaf people in the crowd had perhaps signed with each
other on occasion, though I suspected at the time and later confirmed that they
had never been brought together to interact in any kind of sustained way. This
is not unusual. They all lived twenty minutes or more away from the center of
town in different directions, and in Nepal there seems to be very little sense
among the hearing that deaf people might enjoy or benefit from interacting
with each other. As one father of a deaf teenager put it to me, "What would they
say to each other?" As a general rule, people with disabilities are kept close to
home, and women especially tend to have few opportunities for social engagement beyond their immediate household. Nevertheless, the deaf people present
had been brought together on that day because (I later learned) the VDC chairman had implied that Niraj might help them to access the disability entitle-
ments promised by law but only inconsistently dispersed.

After the designated five minutes had passed, Rina moved to the center
of the impromptu stage and began to address the assembled crowd in sign.
The interpreter, ten feet away in Rina's front left quadrant, dutifully proceeded
to interpret her words. At first, the members of the audience seemed unsure
of where to direct their gaze, shifting quickly back and forth between Rina
and the interpreter. They were obviously unfamiliar with the conventions of
interpreted speech, and consequently for them the event provided a conflicting
set of cues: the sound of the interpreter's voice demanded a certain extent of
attention, but her gaze and demeanor were directed not at those listening to
her but rather inward at Rina. Rina, meanwhile, faced out at the audience and
moved through the most conspicuous parts of the space. I don't know that the
uncertainty ultimately resolved for everyone, but before long all eyes had set-
tled on her. If nothing else, Rina was more visually interesting than the interpreter, who furthermore could be heard without being seen. For the remainder
of the program, the interpreter's voice came from one place, but all bodies were

---

3.   Though "home sign" is the term of choice in the sign language literature (Senghas
     2004; Fusellier-Souza 2006; Brentari et al. 2012), I prefer E. Mara Green's
     "local sign" designation (Green 2012) because it casts the issue in terms of
     scopes of conventionality rather than domestic/public distinctions. Nevertheless,
     I use the term "home sign" here because the phrase (in various translations and
     transliterations) was used occasionally by the deaf Nepalis I spoke to.

focused—collectively and conspicuously—on Rina, someplace else. This effect of displacement is familiar to signers, and they often discussed it in my presence. It must be very frustrating, many commented, for hearing people to never know for sure who is listening to them. How, they wondered, could anyone ever use spoken language discretely?

These considerations of voice and location aside, however, the content of Rina's presentation was itself extremely familiar, built as it was from an only slightly modified version of the political speech genre that characterizes formal discourse in Nepal generally (Hartford 2002; Onta 2006). Rina said that it was with great pleasure that she introduced her esteemed friend Niraj to the respected village community, that she hoped its members would hear her words and reflect upon them, and that the well-being of the deaf was the responsibility of us all. She ended her talk with a familiar rhetorical flourish, proclaiming that the development of NSL must be synonymous with the development of Nepal. As far as political speeches go, there was nothing particularly unusual here save for two facts: first, it was being delivered by a deaf person, and deaf people don't generally give speeches; second, and equally strange, it was being addressed to the five deaf people in the audience, and speeches aren't generally addressed to the deaf. Meanwhile, these five, in addition to comprising only a very small minority of those assembled, understood neither spoken Nepali nor conventional NSL, and as a consequence they gleaned little to nothing of the speech's content. Nevertheless, Rina addressed them as brothers and sisters, far less formally than she addressed others, and she accompanied these identifications with arms outstretched in their direction. At these moments, the deaf visibly acknowledged they were being spoken to, though they seemed distinctly cautious about the sudden appearance of an outsider who could sign.

The effect on the hearing audience members was equally complex but less obvious, organized by the confluence of several simultaneous and often conflicting extents of Rina's intelligibility. Chief among these was the transparency of language. Nobody could understand Rina's signing. It was fast, it was out of sync with the interpreter, and—most importantly—it was in an especially standards-oriented register of NSL. None of the locals had ever learned NSL, but it was nevertheless a surprise to most present that Rina's obvious fluency should manifest so opaquely. Several members of the audience raised this point explicitly to me after the presentation had finished. In the words of one man, "I've never seen anything like that. The language in her hands was so gentle and nice. I liked it. I couldn't understand anything." This irony of too-transparent signing was not lost in the slightest on Rina. As she later explained to me, "Most people only know 'natural' signs, and they think that's what NSL is. When they see signing that they can't understand, they believe it's just empty hand waving." Under more normal circumstances, in other words, deaf opacity suggests an incoherence, one that serves as evidence of deaf minds as vessels filled with more noise than sense. As an exponent of deaf speech, then, Rina, through her own opacity, risked objectification in these terms, and yet other facts of her identity diverted this pattern of uptake. Rina is conspicuously rich, well dressed, and in full command of a hearing employee. She is, ultimately, too obviously well positioned within familiar regimes of power to be easily dismissed as a noisy hand-waving *lāṭo*.

As for the interpreter, the audience understood her better, but perhaps only marginally so. Her spoken Nepali was disorientingly highbrow, composed from a Sanskrit-derived lexicon and assembled together from syntactic templates that were at best unintuitive to speakers of merely vernacular Nepali. This was a Tamang village; though most of the nonelderly adults and school-attending children spoke Nepali fluently, it was nevertheless not their native tongue. Furthermore, as in many other rural parts of Nepal, those most experienced with the pomp of formal speech genres were also the ones most likely to have already migrated away in search of work in Kathmandu, India, or the Arabian peninsula. For those who remained, the linguistic demands at play here sat somewhere between uncomfortable and oppressive. Curiously, however, there was nothing present in the structure of Rina's signing to suggest that it should be translated into spoken Nepali in this way. The long passively voiced sentences, the obscure vocabulary, and the florid metaphors native to development jargon in fact held no analog to anything in the signing being interpreted. NSL does not, for example, divert into Sanskrit loanwords in its highbrow implementations. A rendering in more vernacular Nepali could be equally faithful to Rina's signs, and yet the experience of simpler language would have been very different. I have no reason to believe that the interpreter had colluded with Rina in any way to obscure the content of her translation, and to the contrary it seems just as likely to me that she was unselfconsciously reproducing the genre characteristics of speech giving that seemed most natural to her urban middle-class instincts. Nevertheless, it is extremely conspicuous that Rina chose as her interpreter someone with these rhetorical inclinations and, moreover, that the NFDH and KAD continue to train their interpreters in this way.

Whatever the motivations at stake, this configuration had undeniably powerful consequences for those present. A conspicuously unintelligible speaker was
here generating two very different kinds of opaque speech simultaneously. On
the one hand, the interpreter's spoken language was opaque in exactly the way
that it was expected to be. It exemplified a familiar genre of campaign stump
speeches, royal radio addresses, and government decrees, and thus its rhetorical purpose was clear precisely to the extent that its literal meaning was hard
to recover (Yadava 2007). Power, after all, is familiar as something difficult for
the poor to access. The opacity of Rina's signing was more unexpected, however.
Though the burden of transparency usually falls entirely on the deaf person in
an interaction, Rina's palpable foreignness served to reveal her place in networks
of power and exchange that only infrequently pass through rural Nepal. As a
presence in context, her voice thus emerged from opposite forces: a movement of
hands that was opaque for one reason paired with an interpreted verbal performance that was opaque for a different one. Her signing, thus, was experienced by
the hearing as something unexpectedly unintelligible, forced to remain ambiguously oriented without serious speculation about the contents of her mind. It is
this act of speculation, I believe, that Rina's performance was engineered to cause.

With her half of the presentation complete, Rina acknowledged the VDC
chairman's role in making it possible, and she thanked the village community for
considering her message. She then invited Niraj to address the assembly. As before, the interpreter took her position and voiced Niraj's signing. The signs Niraj
made, however, were very different from the ones Rina had. In contrast to the
furious pace of Rina's natural speech and its twenty-second lead on interpreted
equivalence, Niraj exaggerated his articulations and watched the interpreter
carefully to allow his movements to be matched by her words. The resulting
stream of sign was easily segmented, salient as a series of isolated meanings, and
matched to their real-time re-presentation in far more familiar kinds of Nepali:

- [Hands pressed together]
- *Namaste* (Namaste)
- [Long sweep of index finger spanning audience]
- *tapāiharu* (All of you)
- [Hands brought together repeatedly at tips of fingers]
- *bhetera* (having met)
- [Fingertips close then open at chest]
- *khusi lāgyo* (I feel happy)

- [Points to self]
- *ma* (I)
- [Fingertips cover ear than mouth]
- *bahira hũ* (am deaf)
- [Open hands move in circles]
- *saṃketik bhāṣā* (sign language)
- [Flat hands step up incrementally]
- *bikās* (development)
- [Sweeping circle enclosing all present]
- *hāmi sabaiko* (all of our)
- [Two open hands moving apart]
- *mahatwapurṇa* (important)
- [Right fist pounds left fist]
- *kām* (work)
- [index finger slices through air]
- *ho* (is)

Though the word order here yields a jumbled and choppy English gloss, the Nepali was perfectly fluent and accessible to everyone present: "Namaste. I am happy to meet everyone. I am deaf. The development of sign language is an important job that belongs to us all," and so on. As a further aid to his transparency, Niraj selected his vocabulary carefully to maximize interpretability by nonsigners. For example, to convey the word "important," he actually combined two distinct NSL lexical signs into one coarticulated movement. The first sign, IMPORTANT (figure 10), is far more salient to signers. It combines a relatively arbitrary downward closing of the handshape "म," which represents the first letter of the spoken Nepali word *mahatwapurṇa* ("important"). The second sign, BIG (figure 11), is made by two open hands moving apart in ways far more evocative of the presence of something large. This simultaneity structured a perceptual asymmetry separating the signers and the nonsigners. Though the formal characteristics of BIG were more obviously engaging to the uninitiated audience, the interpreter correctly noticed the more subtle change in handshape and used it to cue the appropriate gloss: *mahatwapurṇa*, "important." While the combination here is effectively redundant, the lamination of the second sign onto the first served to accommodate the hearing expertly. By managing the pace and rhythm through which his movements and meanings were mapped together, Niraj allowed those who witnessed him to deconstruct their relationship in real time, rendering present for all to see a very particular and very carefully crafted part of the landscape of motivations that substantiate his signs.

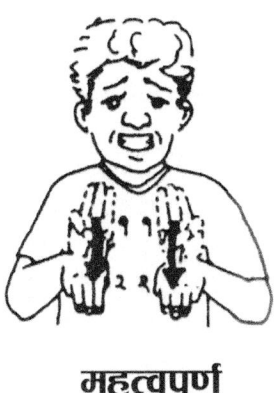

महत्वपूर्ण

Figure 10. IMPORTANT

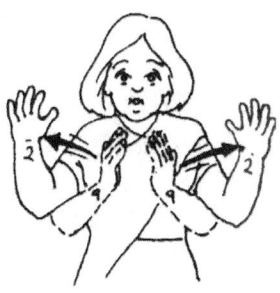

ठूलो

Figure 11. BIG

In this performance, Niraj made himself so transparent to the hearing as to be nearly featureless. As he later explained to me, this technique of self-presentation was part of his broader role in this town. It was intentional, in other words, and made possible by an aptitude for reading the hearing that he had built over the course of many long years. Like many veterans of the program, Niraj characterized his experience of teaching in rural Nepal in ambivalent terms. His lofty idealism was sharply colored by memories of intense and unrelenting boredom during past trips. This is a function, he explained, of who he is in the village. His job is to be radically transparent at all times, and this means having no properties that cannot be read as other than surface phenomena. It means no alignments, no affiliations, no particularity, and no complexity. It means doing his work and going home to sleep afterwards. In service of these ends, his language must always be made general enough to make sense to everybody at all times. It is hard to think of anything more oppressively dull.

Rina, meanwhile, was conspicuously disorienting. The inscrutability of her moving hands was not entirely unexpected, but it ceased to be dismissible as meaningless noise when it came into alignment with her obvious stores of sociopolitical power. At a level of sensible talk, Rina is opaque and Niraj is transparent. In the context of a more broadly pervasive economy of power, however, Rina's familiarity as an important kind of person makes everything previously taken for granted about Niraj feel suddenly very strange. By claiming herself as the more normative signer in this way, Rina renders the question of her opacity suddenly very present to the hearing. One man in the audience was so struck by his experience of her that he later asked if I myself had learned NSL at American college, effectively reframing her language as an expensive and inaccessible kind of expertise. This shift was, I believe, carefully engineered to raise for the hearing the specter of a possibility: what opacity demonstrates is not an absence of deaf interiority but rather a lack of hearing access to it. Perhaps all deaf people, even the ones in this town, have been full of *sense* all along.

As far as subtle manipulations of a crowd go, this was a masterful tandem performance. As I have suggested over the past few chapters, the broadest and most consequential facts of deaf social realities are usually unintelligible to the hearing, but in this village square Niraj and Rina made the hearing feel for the first time that they were *missing* something. Simply by *talking* to each other, they made their audience experience a scope of signing that was not engineered to be transparent specifically for them. The hearing started to feel *hearing*—suddenly, forcefully, and inescapably—and, by feeling hearing, they realized how little access they have to deaf language and deaf ways of organizing the world. In this way, Rina and Niraj have transformed the perception of *absence* into a perception of *opacity*, rendering deaf minds *present* through their inaccessibility to the hearing. They do not try to instruct their audience about what kinds of things deaf minds might contain but instead merely establish the space of possibility for such content. What this intelligibility play creates is an experience of this possibility encountered by the entire village community simultaneously. By opening radical new domains to the engagements of deaf minds, Rina and Niraj have established an entire possible world of deaf things, deaf meanings, deaf experiences, and even deaf politics. They are teaching the hearing how to see the deaf, even and especially when they can't understand them.

Early the next morning, Rina and the interpreter returned to Kathmandu. I stayed with Niraj and observed his classroom for a few days, but after that I too returned to the city. I didn't see Niraj again until he finished his course several months later, but when I did he let me know that he was happy with his outcomes. There were actually six deaf people in the area, as another had been found shortly after the classes began. Three of them ultimately became proficient signers, while one unfortunately was removed from Niraj's reach by her very skeptical father. The remaining two showed signs of primary cognitive impairments that would prevent them from ever participating fully in language, though Niraj was sure that they nevertheless enjoyed attending the class. The hearing attended in significant numbers for the first few weeks, too, but their numbers quickly dropped off because (according to Niraj) the class was too hard and involved homework. One sister of a deaf class member stuck with the material long enough to become an enthusiastic if clumsy signer, however, and Niraj was optimistic that she would be a valuable advocate for the deaf people who would remain in town after he left. In so doing, she may provide an interactive and visible contrast to the "natural" home signs more generally used between the hearing and the deaf. This link will serve to perpetuate the relationship Rina and Niraj so prominently claimed between opaque language and the presence of mind.

THE DEAFNESS OF MOTHERS AND BUILDINGS

One summer afternoon in 2007, roughly sixty deaf activists marched down Thirbam Sadak to Parliament. They were endorsing the candidacy of Raghav Bir Joshi to the Constituent Assembly that would draft Nepal's new constitution, and I had been invited along for what they promised would be a lot of fun. The monsoon skies poured rain upon us, though the only people who really seemed to mind were the members of the rally's ad hoc props committee. For weeks before the event, the committee had worked hard to construct a wide assortment of signs and banners bearing slogans painted in bright colors. As the rain started to fall, the paint began to run, and the paper began to disintegrate. The artists watched as their labor dissolved into bits and pieces washing down into the gutters. Though the rest of the rally kept moving forward without really seeming to notice, the props committee expressed concern that the loss of the signs had undercut the march's purpose completely. There are no bullhorns or audible calls at deaf protests, and as a consequence deaf voice is experienced by the hearing primarily through the alignment of written text and a conspicuous absence of sound. Props are important at deaf political events for the simple reason that they provide the visual cues necessary to alert hearing people to the fact that deaf people are talking. As our leaflets, sandwich boards, signs, and banners dissolved into a pulpy mush, that voice was remanded to scores of marchers signing in a rough approximation of unison: flat hands circling forward, double fingers against ears and then chins, hooked fingers against nostrils, and flat hands against mouths. These signs were inscrutable to the hearing, but like many of the boards before them they all bore a single phrase: "*Sanketik bhāṣā bahiraharuko mātribhāṣā*" (Sign language is the mother language of the deaf).

At face value, this is a strange claim with paradoxical entailments that I am certain were lost on none of the people marching that day. When signers call NSL the "mother language of the deaf" (*Bahira Awaj* 1998), they do so with full, deeply personal, and often fraught awareness of the fact that most of their mothers do not actually know the language. This is no small circumstance. The disjunction that deafness can create between hearing mothers and their deaf children is perhaps the most basic ground of the deaf experience. It carves a rift in one of humanity's most important vectors of socialization—the linguistic connection between parent and child—imposing on deaf Nepal what is often a devastating isolation. If there is one fact that is constantly and conspicuously present to deaf fields of experience, it is that language is not something to be taken for granted as shared with anyone. The public does not sign, and families sign often least of all. To talk then of deaf mother languages reveals an unorthodox way of constituting the truth of these kinds of statements.

For the hearing, the possibility of a deaf mother language builds on a very different semantic slippage: to unfamiliar encounters with these slogans, it is not at all clear whether sign language *should be* the mother language of the deaf or whether perhaps it *already is*. Such ambiguities are familiar to politics generally, but here I think the logic of political instruction was intended to be more indirect. As one protester explained: "They look at us and just see hands moving.

We look at them and just see lips moving. But, here, we meet in the middle; for a moment, we're the same. And, suddenly, they understand." The question of *what* they understand is quite a bit more complicated, but the possibility of the transformation it engineers comes down to the power of deaf people in groups. Even without the signs and banners, the sight of an exuberant crowd signing in unison serves to displace the category of deafness away from generalized encounters with *lāṭohood* and onto the fact of a self-engaged deaf community acting in a particular place and time. What this protest accomplished, in other words, was to get the hearing to *look* at something that normally only deaf people see.[4]

Deafness, like all social categories, is built from a history of conflict and contestation, but what I find more interesting here is the way that these categories allow the deaf and the hearing to share an experience of something present together. Kinship, in this sense, is not a naïve descriptive fact but rather a template for recognition that deaf social practices operationalize or flout in order to strategically craft a world of things apparent to the hearing. The question of mother languages in particular lays bare the most familiar dynamic of group boundary making as it runs together and falls apart within the biographies of deaf individuals. In these moments, deaf lives are built from the unfamiliar unions and disjunctions of too familiar categories (cf. Rapp and Ginsburg 2011, or "analogies", in Strathern's language [Strathern 2011]).

For all these reasons, we must be especially cautious when applying familiar cultural logics to the deaf. When we see, for example, the highly ritualized ways in which deaf communities in many parts of the world grant signed names to new members (Lane, Hoffmeister, and Bahan 1996), it is very tempting to understand these acts as constituting a rebaptism of sorts. In these terms, we might understand deaf communities as a kind of neokinship, counterposing the entailments of the hearing. Throughout this book, however, I argue that these

---

4.   This strategy of commensuration through shared acts of sight has deep roots in South Asia. As Robert Desjarlais discusses in his excellent work *Sensory Biographies*, perception is experienced in at least some contexts in Nepal not as a *reception* of external stimuli but rather as an extension of the self into the thing being experienced. In the words of Desjarlais's principal interlocutor, Ghang Lama, "The sem [a Yolmo term with analogs in many Nepali languages that Desjarlais translates as "heartmind"] goes to the object seen, meets it, and then brings back to the person an image of the thing seen" (Desjarlais 2003, 57). A great deal of Hindu and Buddhist iconography, likewise, is elaborated around the premise that to see something is to "blend" oneself with the thing seen (Jhala 1997).

oppositions and purifications neglect the extent to which the hearing world's architectures remain present to deaf personal experience. If deaf spaces house a culture and deaf communities define a kinship, we must remember that both ultimately keep bankers' hours. At 5:00 p.m., when the offices close and Thirbam Sadak starts to clear out, deaf people *go home*.

In precisely these terms, the question of disability is critical to contemporary anthropology because it reveals the extent to which cultural expectations accumulate in the worlds that people build (Hansen and Philo 2007; Macpherson 2010). Deaf difference in particular is often hidden by the formal shape of the categories imposed on its actors, institutions, and practices. It is this experience perhaps, more than any question of identity, that unifies the disabled. Curbs, for example, are both created by and essentially invisible to those not in wheelchairs. Their material substance—a mere four inches of raised concrete—underdetermines and even obscures the radically different kinds of entailments they impose on feet and wheels. They were designed not to route or hinder the movement of any particular class of people but merely to manage far more mundane issues of water drainage. Nevertheless, they fill the world with accidental effects that shape the landscape profoundly for some but not others (cf. Friedner and Osborne 2013). These effects are intelligible only from very particular subject positions.

Thirbam Sadak is where the deaf are, but to be reminded that it is not simply a deaf space we need look no further than the dynamics of its vehicles and pedestrians. The road—narrow, busy, and paved right up to the steps of the shops and houses on it—is shared among a wide diversity of participants, human and otherwise, but amidst this diversity there is no doubt that cars have claimed the right of way. The uneasy truce that stands is built both by and for the hearing. Cars blare their horns as they streak down the road and pedestrians get out of the way at the sound of them. This is a very salient architecture of the senses for those who cannot hear. Car horns don't exist as sound for deaf pedestrians, and there is no clear logic by which car drivers can recognize the deaf as such. When I asked deaf people what was hard about being deaf, likewise, "not being able to hear car horns" always made the shortlist alongside more obviously political concerns about social and linguistic isolation, ideological oppression, stigmatization, and limited access to public institutions. In its hidden logics of organization, the landscape fails the deaf in ways that the hearing only rarely come to notice.

In Kathmandu broadly, there is perhaps no better example of everything that goes unnoticed in the present than the sedimentations that constitute the city streets along which the mother language protest marched. Though various authorities have over the years imposed their particular organizational schemes on the area around Thirbam Sadak (Slusser 1982; Pant and Funo 2003), other generations have simply built on top of what was already there. The resultant legacies of architecture stand as echoes of plans and people long since dead, erased as coherent narratives but nevertheless still consequential as fragments of stone and sod. What used to be parade grounds are now tracks for joggers, and what used to be palace gardens are now open fields for young couples and cows to wander through. Though these legacies are rarely intelligible in narrative terms, they are nevertheless consequential for how they shape space.

The landscape around Thirbam Sadak is dominated by feudal-era palaces, open-air workshops, and a brand-new five-story shopping arcade. For visitors and locals alike, these juxtapositions are often described as evidence of the rapid and dramatic changes currently taking place in Nepal. There is, of course, a great deal that has changed, but in other terms this space could just as easily be a story about continuity. The area was a favorite residential quarter for extended members of the Rana political regime (1846–1951), and it is still considered a "nice" part of town. Though property here is extremely valuable, the complexity of contemporary land tenure has also rendered it relatively illiquid. What stands is therefore patchy: some lots sit wide open and empty as they await development by cash-poor or legally encumbered owners, while others are built to claustrophobic density. It is not uncommon to see buildings that have been literally sawed in half along a vertical axis, the strikingly visual artifact of disputes among brothers as they divide up the already divided inheritances of their fathers and grandfathers.

To the inhabitants of the area, the crumbling mansions are "old" and the glitzy apartment buildings are "new," but this sorting establishes one narrative of history while erasing another. Though bricks and mortar may represent a time superseded by steel and glass, the once magnificent walls are just as contemporary in their present state of decay as they were when they were built. Indeed, the walls are crumbling not because they are old but rather because of how their owners have come to occupy the new organizations of the urban economy. To the fading aristocrats living in dilapidated mansions and their better-positioned cousins building apartment towers, the continuity or discontinuity of power is simply a matter of where you stand.[5] The architecture here is a perfect

---

5.   See A. A. Johnson (2013) for a parallel account of the intuitive entanglements of landscape and change in Thailand.

composite, built from stone and clay but existent as it is because of a vastly larger confluence of histories.

Every Friday, deaf people converge in large numbers on Thirbam Sadak to add their own contributions to this history. The formal culmination of this event each week is a series of speeches and announcements given at KAD by members of the elected board. This includes useful practical information about ceremonies, picnics, projects, and protests, but as a matter of tradition it also incorporates field reports compiled by deaf emissaries sent into the hearing world to seek out information on a wide range of themes in general knowledge. One week, for example, a board member reported on his meeting with the head of Kathmandu's premier medical school, where he ostensibly (though definitely not actually) learned for the first time that smoking is hazardous to one's health. A few weeks earlier, another board member presented on the legalities of music piracy. Though these presentations are usually very brief, often less than five minutes, themes deemed particularly important are sometimes extended into day-long conferences organized by KAD. One conference I attended dealt exclusively with the pleasures and hazards of romantic love, and another one was dedicated to earthquake preparedness. Regardless of topic, the purpose is always explicitly pedagogical.

When I asked members of the board why they allotted so much community face time to matters of what they called "GK" (general knowledge), they unanimously agreed that they did so because it was necessary. Even general facts are not to be taken for granted in deaf populations, they said, because the forms of information and intuition that generally accrue in the course of normal socialization often come and go without deliberate transmission, emergent instead from accidental patterns of overhearing that systematically exclude the deaf (Ochs and Shohet 2006; Kimmel 2008). This space of gaps can include highly charged topics like sex, abuse, health, and morality, but also more technical things like how to open a bank account, what to do if there's a fire, and where to buy fresh produce. By offering this general knowledge in explicitly formal ways, then, KAD seeks to establish itself as a primary site of deaf socialization.

There is, however, quite a bit more to this story. Though these presentations without fail maintain an overtly instrumental logic, they are at the same time addressed conspicuously often to an audience that is entirely absent. The earthquake conference, for example, included a long presentation by a prominent deaf signer on how to maximize seismic resistance when manufacturing concrete. Though the information offered was (as far as I could tell) technically rigorous, it presumed a skill set, means of production, and domain of practice that none of the participants even loosely possessed. There just aren't any deaf-run cement factories. Even talks on more basic matters often exclude exactly the people who need them. The majority of KAD's regular members have been attending these events for years, and any among them who need to buy vegetables already know where to do it. Recent migrants into the Kathmandu deaf scene might certainly lack this knowledge, but as a rule they also lack the sophistication with NSL necessary to follow the fluent signing in which it is presented. Precisely by virtue of needing this information, they are unable to hear it. Though socializing these newly arrived deaf people is indeed a basic function of KAD, in practice the bulk of this work happens in quieter and more intimate settings. During the presentations designed ostensibly for them, these new arrivals tend instead to stand quietly to the side, watching the crowd more than the speaker, while everyone else tries hard to seem engaged while playing discreetly with their cell phones. Though there is widespread agreement that these presentations are important, it is not at all clear that the information they present is meant to be *useful* to the people there to obtain it. Instead, they seem to orchestrate what is primarily an aesthetic effect. Mainstream discourse networks often rely on architectures of perception that marginalize the deaf, and deaf knowledge is most often systematically inaccessible to the hearing. As a response, perhaps, these performances reconstitute hearing expertise through deaf ways of telling, thereby establishing KAD and other such community spaces as a point of origin for deaf ways of knowing.

At other moments, these vectors of telling are conspicuously reversed. At formal deaf events, for example, interpreters are often granted an unusual degree of prominence, even and especially when there are no hearing people in the audience. When delivering speeches, deaf community members will sometimes speak from the periphery of the stage, their backs turned to the audience to face an interpreter watching. They are in these moments effectively unhearable, their words invisible but redelivered by interpreters using spoken Nepali from a microphone front and center. These spatial configurations offer a stark counterpoint to those engineered by Rina and Niraj in Rasuwa District earlier in this chapter. There, signers used space to foreground the (un)intelligibility of signing as a genred discursive act, and by contrast these other arrangements seem strangely self-effacing. They appear to imagine a world in which signing is subordinate to speech, even in the absence of hearing people to hear it.[6] When I

6. Notably, these same dynamics do not occur when speech-to-speech translations are used at hearing events. When translating from Nepali to English, for example,

asked organizers why the interpreters were given the most visible spot while the entire audience was forced to squint into the wings, however, my question was usually met with an appeal to scale. There are, by any metric, a far greater number of people in Nepal who speak Nepali than who know NSL, and it makes sense to prioritize the channel that can reach the greatest audience. The fact that there were few or none of these Nepali speakers present seemed ultimately beside the point. Instead, in these moments, the deaf community seeks to address a public most broadly defined. There may be no deaf concrete manufacturers ready to assimilate earthquake tips nor any hearing audience members to benefit from interpreters at center-stage, but nevertheless constituting and participating in an anonymous deaf-plus-hearing public means reclaiming the possibility that there *might* be (cf. Debenport 2013). To this end, there is something very powerful about passing hearing things through deaf voices and deaf things through hearing voices. According to a cultural framework that values history over form, managing circulation offers a powerful basis of group participation.

A few years after the primary fieldwork for this book was completed, KAD secured a new location just up the road from the site it had occupied for decades. To any casual observer, this new site was unambiguously superior to the old. It featured multiple private offices, ample classroom space, and a sunny, wide open floor plan oriented around a large central courtyard. It was and is a truly beautiful space, offering a sharp experience of contrast to everyone who remembers the dark, dank, and cramped quarters of the old site. Though KAD's leaders admitted some anxiety at the time about the cost of their new lease (particularly to the extent that it expands their dependency on the British and Swedish deaf organizations that partially subsidize their programs), there was never any question for them that this move was necessary for the continued maturation of deaf political activism. This is an important claim. Though the prestige of having a space that doesn't smell like a sewer every time it rains was no doubt part of the choice to move, the real transformation at stake remains hidden in the implications of angles and architecture.

There is a rich literature on the mediation of voice in minority and disability (see Gerber 1990; Das and Addlakha 2001; Bagatell 2007; or, most literally,

---

interpreters will usually stand to the side of the main stage, or if possible even behind the audience. When NSL interpreters are hired to work at hearing events, likewise, they will usually stand far from the podium and as close as possible to the deaf people present.

Wickenden 2011), but nowhere is the problem of speech mechanics so easily noticed as with the deaf. In hearing worlds, speech is organized by dynamics of proximity. Distance creates boundaries of inaudibility, and technologies like the loudspeaker overcome this hindrance by reconstituting voice simultaneously everywhere and nowhere (Warner 2002). For the deaf, however, the politics of voice unfolds in very different terms as a micropolitics of obstruction, of breaks in lines of sight and limited fields of vision. The world's spaces were built to accommodate voice as sound but only very rarely as scattered vectors of light. This unstated orientation is revealed in the placement of pillars, the design of doors, and the shape of rooms. A building built by deaf people would begin with very different principles. Though still not perfect, KAD's new office space was substantially better suited to deaf mechanics of talk, and it was for this reason more than anything else that the old space was replaced. The wide open court-yard in particular, I was told, would lay the foundation for a mature deaf politics because it allows everyone to see everyone else at the same time. Conversations can now happen with participants standing in a circle of mutual visibility, rather than packed into a crowded room where some must inevitably hold their backs to others. This matters because, for the deaf, the limits of simultaneous discourse are a function of the number of people who can see each other at once.

Not everyone was thrilled with the new space, however. The move happened quickly, and, according to critics, the decision to make it received insufficient public scrutiny. I had already returned to Chicago by this point, but actors on both sides of the conversation wrote to me with obvious seething frustration. This was certainly not the first time I'd heard complaints about a KAD board (or, conversely, complaints by a board about the unrealistic expectations of the KAD membership), but the tone here was more vitriolic than anything I'd ever experienced, dividing the deaf community along a fault-line previously hidden. To soothe the tensions, the elected leadership tried to explain that this new en-vironment was proof of everything that the deaf had achieved over the last three decades. In response, others suggested to me that the new building represented a total capitulation to hearing mindsets. I'll admit that I loved the new KAD site as soon as I saw it later that year, and it was hard for me to understand how anyone could object to it. I spent more than a thousand hours in the old office building, and it was always morosely uncomfortable. It was cold in the winter and rank in the summer, and the bugs were often relentless. Simply being there too long seemed to make everyone grumpy. The new space, in contrast, is beau-tiful, and on a sunny day it is an eminently pleasant place to pass an afternoon.

My first thought upon seeing it was that I'd wished the move had happened before I'd ever arrived. This wish was most tangibly driven by memories of discomfort, but there was a professional dimension here too. The old KAD site was dominated by awkward corners and unexpected staircases. These noisy contours made it difficult for me as an anthropologist to observe what was going on in anything more than a narrow sliver of space at any given moment. But, as I was later told by a deaf friend close enough for frank talk, this was exactly the point. The fact that I saw it all as a defect was clear evidence that I was hearing. I don't think this was meant as an admonition so much as a simple affirmation of fact: the world is filled with things that are visible to some but not to others, and I couldn't see the problem with the new office for the same reason that the colorblind can't see certain contrasts of hue.

The problem with the new KAD space is precisely that everyone can see everyone else at all times, and to understand why this is undesirable to some requires a deeply felt enmeshment in the coherences of deaf life. At the old site, conversations were necessarily intimate and private. It was hard to hold a meeting involving more than twenty people at once, so as a consequence the dissemination of information across the deaf community was necessarily mediated by a wide and distributed network of relays. Things became known or remained unknown because of nuanced practices of social exchange with relatively few central nodes or single points of failure. Being able to see everyone at the same time obliterates these very deaf engagements with privacy, knowledge, communication, and interdependency. The new office makes everything known because it makes everything seeable at once, reorganizing the intelligibility of the deaf community as a function of normative form rather than social history. This alignment of vision elides the processes by which things come to be in social place, and it makes it easy to forget that objects are made by the subjects who engage them. To a group of people whose political sensibility is organized around exactly these kinds of dynamics, a place in which everyone can see everyone else at once is effacing.

This notion that deaf values can be implicit in something like architectural form is critically important to an anthropology of the deaf. It reflects significantly on Frank Bechter's concept of the "convert culture" (Bechter 2008, 2009). In his remarkable study of American deaf narrative genres, Bechter demonstrates that deaf storytelling is structurally organized by shifts of narrative perspective, encouraging people to view nondeaf contexts through deaf subaltern lenses (via Spivak 1988). This emphasis on perspective shifting is about the manifestation of what Bechter calls "trapped value": relationships in the world that are invisible until they are disentangled from normative structures of meaning. In these terms, what is missing from the new KAD is deaf *sense*. In the first chapter, I defined *sense* as a local intuition about how it is that objects are experienced as copresent with the people, contexts, and histories that brought them to be. For a thing to have *sense* is to say that it is more than it appears. This attention to the history of things is central to deaf activism broadly, and the problem with the new KAD is that its architecture conspires against these modes of attention experienced by members as so essential to deaf social practices. Very simply, some allege, the new building doesn't allow things to be put in deaf terms. These concerns about social and material architectures were presented to members of the board, and most acknowledged the problem. But they then went on to say that it was time for the deaf community to look forward, not back. To this, one particularly vocal critic responded: "That's a very hearing thing to say."

LOREM IPSUM

Shanta Raj Shrestha, a deaf member of KAD whose name I've changed at his request, is a self-described computer enthusiast. For a period of about six months in 2008, the focus of his enthusiasm was the *Lorem Ipsum* generator he discovered on his laptop. He called this tool (only somewhat glibly) "the greatest achievement of science," and with an almost evangelical zeal he worked to share *Lorem Ipsum* with anyone he could.

For those whose lives have heretofore lacked *Lorem Ipsum* and thus might wonder what gets generated by a *Lorem Ipsum* generator, the answer is blocks of text like this:

> Lorem ipsum dolor sit amet, consectetur adipisicing elit, sed do eiusmod tempor incididunt ut labore et dolore magna aliqua. Ut enim ad minim veniam, quis nostrud exercitation ullamco laboris nisi ut aliquip ex ea commodo consequat. Duis aute irure dolor in reprehenderit in voluptate velit esse cillum dolore eu fugiat nulla pariatur. Excepteur sint occaecat cupidatat non proident, sunt in culpa qui officia deserunt mollit anim id est laborum.

Lorem Ipsum is nonsense, a jabberwocky of pseudo-Latin cribbed five hundred years ago from a mangled bit of Cicero. In functional terms, *Lorem Ipsum* is *filler* text, and the name "*Lorem Ipsum*" refers generally to both the particular filler text quoted above and the genre of filler texts more generally.

The practice of populating documents with *Lorem Ipsum*—called "Greeking" (as in, "It's Greek to me")—has important applications in the design industry. When setting typefaces or page layouts, designers will often populate templates with *Lorem Ipsum* to showcase their work. This is a response to a very particular problem in publishing: when demonstrating visual components, designers often find themselves wrestling with the latent power of text to communicate, even when the particularities of its subject matter are ostensibly irrelevant. Though I might instruct a reader to notice only the shape of the letter "c" in "cat," the word nevertheless will tend to invoke an experienced presence of the furry creature. For the purposes of visual design, this is distracting at best and alienating at worst. Cats, like everything else, carry with them in context vast tangles of association that are neither controlled nor even fully seen by any particular individual. If my reader is a potential customer who happens to loathe small domestic animals, this incidental meaning might cost me a sale. In the course of normal language use, it is tremendously difficult to exhibit form without content, and *Lorem Ipsum* was designed in hopes of offering a way around this problem.

Lorem Ipsum acquired its canonical form through a series of happy accidents. It began as a passage of actual Latin, but over time it accumulated errors made by manual typesetters who tried to recreate it without any knowledge of what it meant. Over the course of this centuries-long game of telephone, it became something that *looks like* language without actually *being* language. To this same end, *Lorem Ipsum* generators use variously sophisticated algorithms to produce gibberish that can look real without actually *meaning* anything. This process will generally involve heuristics to distribute common and rare letters appropriately, phonological sensitivities that ensure natural syllable shapes, and word- and sentence-length constraints that make the language "feel" right. There are *Lorem Ipsum* generators for Latin, English, German, Hindi, and any number of other languages, which produce texts that look like these languages without actually bearing a semantic content. These are statistically well-formed words and sentences that aren't actually words and sentences.

Shanta Raj discovered the *Lorem Ipsum* generator in the spring of 2008, buried deep in the submenus of a popular webpage layout application he had purchased. To most of the world outside of the publishing industry, *Lorem Ipsum* is at most a novelty. Shanta Raj found it fascinating, important, and hilarious, however, and he proceeded to incorporate it into his daily life. He filled every desktop publishing template he could find with *Lorem Ipsum* text and printed them out with a degree of care that can only be called tender. He made impeccably formatted dispatches on official letterheads, flashy newsletters with high-concept designs, and long rambling walls of text signed with his own name at the bottom in blue ink. He designed preaddressed envelopes and business cards, pages and pages of magazine articles spliced with stock images, and even a properly formatted will of last testament. All of it was carefully formatted gibberish. Shanta Raj even made a fake newspaper, paid to have it printed on authentic tabloid stock, and proceeded to travel about the city reading it in public. He made *Lorem Ipsum* posts on his Facebook page, and even opened a new account just for *Lorem Ipsum* content. He then proceeded to friend this account to every celebrity and public company he could think of just to post on their walls. For a period of around six months, he seemed intent on filling the world with filler.

When I asked Shanta Raj to explain his interest in *Lorem Ipsum*, he made it very clear that he found my questions tedious. This was an elaborate practical joke, he explained, and the humor inherent in the performance should be self-evident. By asking him to explain everything, I was ruining it. Though he was perfectly accurate to point out how clumsy my intuitions were, I think he felt bad about it after the fact because the next day he invited me to venture out from the office with him to see how this whole thing worked. We rode the bus reading fake newspapers, we handed out fake business cards with fake job titles, we distributed fake political leaflets with fake party logos and fake demands for change, and we dropped fake letters bearing fake news from fake loved ones into real residential mail slots.

For the people we encountered, our texts were deeply confusing. Shanta Raj noticed this, pointed it out, and took considerable delight in the fact that it was happening. This was, I think, the whole point. People attributed the presence of meaning to Shanta Raj's texts because they looked like the kinds of things that *should* be meaningful. After all, we were reading them, we were encouraging others to read them, and we had spent the time and money to have them properly printed. They demanded attention in all normative semiotic channels because, ultimately, that is what text genres are supposed to do. But, Shanta Raj's texts were never meant to be intelligible for denotative content. They served instead to draw his public into a cargo cult of conflated real things and fake things, thereby invoking the ambiguous power of each. They exist not to be meaningful but rather to showcase the problem of meaningfulness itself.

Because language is the material basis and most conspicuous mode of deaf difference, it is no surprise that deaf intelligibility is often staked on specifically linguistic questions. The precise contours here are complex and important. In the context of deaf Nepal, language is—among other things—often quite fun, but playful engagements between the deaf and the hearing are particularly wrought with investments of knowledge, meaning, and power. Perhaps because the deaf are significantly dispossessed of the "productive" worlds of work and talk, shared entertainments are often remembered in particularly light-hearted terms by the hearing. In my interviews, hearing siblings would often recall the games they used to play with their deaf brothers and sisters before anything else. One sister even went so far as to say that *guccho*—a traditional village game of flinging pebbles—actually *was* her brother's language. This is a far more vivid encounter than the ones she used to describe her other siblings, in which the relationship was characterized by more abstract notions of purpose, obligation, need, caring for or being cared for, and so on. Kinship is especially overdetermined by logics of apparent necessity, and this makes playful exchanges particularly expressive of cultural aspirations. Play, that which is by definition not necessary, is freer to express. Shanta Raj characterized his interest in *Lorem Ipsum* first and foremost as a chance for fun, but the sheer scale of pleasure he derived from this kind of play demonstrates its importance as work.

In these terms, I would suggest that his engagement with *Lorem Ipsum* is quintessentially deaf. The punchline to the joke here, I think, is how painfully easy it is to mistake form for content and vice versa. More importantly, this fact of conflation itself reveals something fundamentally critical about the social histories necessary to make form and content appear distinct and dyadic in the first place. The sheer scope of institutional function that is necessary for simple ink marks on a piece of paper to carry meaning is simply staggering. It requires an entire history of writing and a community connected by it. As a deaf man engaged in deaf advocacy, Shanta Raj is constantly aware of this vastness of social history, and with his *Lorem Ipsum* texts he is thrusting the same experience onto the hearing. This is a joke with deeply pedagogical intentions. What Shanta Raj knows, and what the hearing usually don't, is that people are so invested in first-order articulations of form and content that they fail to experience the higher organizational frames that make the very fact of association possible in the first place. As a hearing person, I didn't get the joke without a laborious demonstration, and that is exactly the point; Shanta Raj's deaf friends, on the other hand, found it funny immediately.

When you're deaf, everybody thinks you don't have *sense*, though of course you do. It seems no coincidence, then, that Shanta Raj takes such pleasure in filling the world with objects that everybody assumes have *sense*, when in fact they don't. Objects are easily mistaken as independent of the subjects who engage them, and being able to manage this possibility is a subtle and tremendous power. Shanta Raj is a connoisseur of these asymmetries, and his ability to export them from deaf contexts to the hearing world expresses an especially playful version of the kinds of mastery at the core of deaf politics. In his project, he reveals a sensitivity to a dimension of being that is usually taken for granted, and in these terms deaf political value is assembled at the invisible interstices of hearing perception. If we track these interventions, we begin to see how the practices of intelligibility mobilized by deaf activists serve to invoke and constitute a history of deaf things in hearing places.

INTELLIGIBILITY REPLAY

A few weeks after I returned to Kathmandu from my trip to Rasuwa with Niraj and Rina, Rina texted me to say that the one-act play she had been rehearsing would be exhibited soon as street theater. I had no idea that she had been working on anything, though I knew she had an interest in acting. I had seen her perform several times in the past, mostly in pieces that were sophisticated but very difficult for me to follow, in an abstract expressionist kind of way. This new show was scheduled to premiere just before dusk at Kathmandu's Durbar Square, an ancient temple and palace complex adjacent to the popular New Road shopping district. The area was particularly busy that day, and before the show began an enthusiastic crew gathered together a large crowd of curious onlookers. I'll admit that I was expecting another allegory about hearing oppression, filled with symbolism so oblique that few would understand any of it. Much to my surprise, however, the piece Rina and her collaborators performed that day was nothing less than a pitch-perfect recreation of her presentation with Niraj in the village square just a few weeks earlier. It included everything except me: the interpreter, the stop for lunch, the contrastive forms of signing, the extension of deaf villagers into kinship categories, and the conspicuous use of translation or nontranslation to create managed effects of opacity. The critical difference, of course, was that this was an explicit re-presentation: urban residents of Kathmandu assembled to watch Rina speak not to *them* but rather to carefully assembled caricatures of village inhabitants (cf. Briggs 2003). This was a displacement, in other words, of an overt act of teaching *there* into something that ostensibly went without saying *here*, with the invisibilities and misrecognitions that took place in that village square offered as emblems of everything backwards. To the affluent shoppers who stopped to watch, this performance thus came with a wink and a nudge: "We don't need to tell *you* any of this, do we?" It was a clear and instructive parable of how to avoid the very foolish mistake of not seeing the deaf.

When you're deaf, very little can be taken for granted about what the hearing know about you, and as a consequence deaf political interventions are most often organized around broadly pedagogical attempts to remind the hearing that they should think about what they take for granted too. Through a broad range of interventions—macro- and micro-, interactive and architectural, serious and silly—the deaf are teaching the hearing how to see. As a logic of social action, this plays out as a perpetual second-orderness, a metaorientation to the dynamics of notice that make things present in the world. Where the hearing are attentive to a particular thing, the deaf must be attentive to the order of social facts one step abstracted from that thing. Where, for example, the hearing are ambivalent about the visibility of deafness, the deaf are crafting games about visual ambivalence. Where sign language is mistaken for a more general gestural habitus, the deaf seek mastery over the formal properties that make signing more or less distinctively salient. Where the hearing try to understand printed language, the deaf organize elaborate practical jokes about the conditions of possibility behind print. These asymmetries of salience and invisibility, of manifestation and disappearance, appear as a movement between semiotic and epistemological regimes: a metasemiosis that appears as semiosis, an epistemology that appears as knowledge, and a process that appears as form. Deaf politics, in short, is a particular way of making the vastness of deaf worlds intelligible—or not.

The deaf can claim no particular monopoly over these techniques, though I find their intuitions about the cultural organization of perception instructive. The hearing manage a world of things sensibly present too, of course, though at least on the matters relevant to this ethnography they tend to be quite a bit more absent-minded about it. In this book, I have framed *intelligibility* as an explicitly ethnographic basis of critical methodology, but the theory I propose is at its core a reformulation of these distinctly deaf responses to problems of perception and objecthood. In this sense, this entire project should be understood as an elaboration and reframing of deaf cultural knowledge. Beginning with the premise that philosophy and cultural intuition are separated only by genre and pedigree, this chapter thus argues that Nepali deaf communities—in their social sensibilities, in their political projects, and in their aesthetics of expression—present important and innovative answers to the very old problem of what it means to say that difference is constituted in context. By intervening in the way that the hearing public encounters the objects of its own perceptions, the deaf teach the hearing to see a world that is kinder to deaf lives.

In *The Gender of the Gift*, Marilyn Strathern famously argued that radical social theory and radical political action might be fundamentally incompatible ambitions. This is ultimately a question of categories:

> So two radicalisms emerge: (1) a radical politics: concerned to change our own condition, we see it in the condition of others too, and seek for change wherever we encounter persons like ourselves; and (2) a radical scholarship, which questions the grounds upon which identity is constructed or conditions shared. Changing the way one thinks may or may not be regarded as practical action, but academic radicalism often appears to result in otherwise conservative action or nonaction. Radical politics, in turn, has to be conceptually conservative. That is, its job is to operationalize already understood concepts or categories, such as "equality" or "men." It is in the radical nature of much feminist scholarship that potential lies for anthropological scholarship, but the field of or context for feminist debate itself (women's oppression) entails the activation of conceptually conservative constructs with which anthropologists may too easily lose patience. (Strathern 1988, 27)

What I would like to suggest is that the deaf have found an innovative way around this dilemma, one with deeply instructive relevance to communities of all sorts. When deaf people and hearing people engage over the coexperience of something, they maintain dramatically different extents of awareness about what those objects contain and what situates them as present in social context. In recognizing these asymmetries, the deaf build spaces of unexpected value in the interstices of what the hearing see, occupying the categories available to them without ever losing sight of the fact that these categories emerge from social histories far too easily forgotten. This is the constitution of deaf difference, at least in its most critical orientation. What the deaf have accomplished in this regard is a logic of social being that escapes the limits imposed by models of personal identity (compare recent work in postleft anarchism, e.g., Landstreicher 2002). In a world that too often imagines itself to have left the question of culture behind, this space of difference hosts the potential of radical change. Seeing it, however, requires careful alignments of ethnographic attention.

CHAPTER 5

Citing signs

विद्याऽविद्याप्रविभगरुपं अप्रविभगं /
कालभेददर्शनाऽभ्यासेन मूर्तिविभागभावनया च //
. . . ब्रह्मेति प्रतिज्ञायते /
न हि //

Speech's form appears distinguishable into parts through knowledge, but in itself—as it is—no distinctions exist. Seeing is a habit acquired in time, and our habits impose on sight the idea that forms are made up from parts. . . . This is how reality is known. But, it is not so.

– Bhartṛhari, *Vākyapadīya 1.1 vṛtti*

THE ICONIC AND THE ARBITRARY . . .

In spoken languages, the sound patterns of words tend to be arbitrary, but it is at least conceivable that things could have been otherwise. We might, for example, identify different species of birds by reproducing their calls, or we might use modulations of vowel length to distinguish between small dogs and large dooooooogs. We might, in other words, have all come to speak languages so transparently evocative that Charles Hockett could never have claimed, as he famously did, that the *duality of patterning* is a design feature of human language (Hockett 1960). As far as the axioms of linguistics go, this is an important one.

In simplest terms, the duality of patterning suggests that all meaningful units of language are themselves composed from a fixed inventory of essentially meaningless atomic elements. Language, to this way of thinking about it, is more like Lego than clay. A word like "cat," for example, refers to a class of domesticated animals as a holistic sound, but it is at the same time realized in speech as a sequence of discrete acoustic categories that are themselves meaningless—/k/, /æ/, and /t/. When setting out to describe a given language for the first time, linguists devote tremendous effort to identifying these units of composition and mapping their limits. There is great benefit to be had in doing so. By postulating that every conceivable utterance in a given language is built from a fixed set of consonants and vowels, speech becomes a thing that can be broken into its component parts. We can abstract it away from the messy realities of everyday use, discovering in its place a powerful formalism to define it. As an academic discipline, modern linguistics is built on the premise of this tier of organization.

Describing the sounds of language is always a challenging task, however, because the particular ways in which particular languages draw boundaries around their categories of sound serve to shape a landscape of linguistic perception, the contours of which largely determine what speakers are and aren't able to hear. Spoken Nepali has four distinct sounds that English speakers tend to identify equivalently as "t," for example, and most Nepalis meanwhile have a relatively hard time hearing a difference between the names "Jack" and "Zack." Nevertheless, even as these perceptual habits shape how language is and isn't heard, speakers have often very little awareness of them. In context, language is substantiated by intricate particularities of sound, and yet these particularities themselves are rarely intelligible to the people who use it. There is nothing especially /k/-like about cats, for example, and a *cat* is not expected to be more similar to a *hat* than to a *dog* simply on the basis of acoustic similarity alone. Speakers likewise cannot produce a sound exactly halfway between "hat" and "cat" and reasonably hope it will be understood to indicate some kind of hybrid: a rodent-chasing mammal worn on the head during cold weather, for example. There are notable exceptions to this—smog, sporks, mocktails, and tofurkeys come to mind—but for the most part it certainly seems that the duality of patterning holds true. The meaning of words and the material properties of sounds are, by and large, very separate things.[1]

---

1.   There is a fascinating literature on ideophones (see especially Alpher 2001; Voeltz and Kilian-Hatz 2001) that demonstrates the limits of arbitrariness in spoken

This expectation of arbitrariness has vexed signers for as far back as the recorded histories go (Defoe 1720; Buffon 1801). Though the *efficacy* of signing as a communicative practice has been noted by observers for centuries,[2] it was not until the 1960s that signed languages were first recognized in the modern West as *languages* in any rigorous sense (Stokoe 1960; Sacks 1989). Ironically, it was the very fact of their efficacy—experienced by nonsigners as an immediacy at odds with the usual opacity of linguistic convention—that served to undermine their larger status for so many years. So long as signing appeared motivated by pantomime and other nonlinguistic sensibilities, there seemed to be little need to explain it further. These expectations were ruptured dramatically during the sign language boom of the 1960s and 1970s, and since that time the linguistic study of deaf communities has produced a wealth of high-quality work.[3] In the course of this transformation, however, the driving trend in research has been to reclaim signed languages for linguistic analysis by finding within them analogs to the dually patterned categories of speech. Signs may not exhibit a structural relationship between consonants and vowels, for example, but nevertheless there do appear to be real constraints on the lexical syllable shape they have, such as strong tendencies for certain kinds of symmetry in two-handed signs. Implicit in these observations has been an attempt to justify the linguistic status of sign *against* its apparent iconicity of form. Even when signing appears gestural, this argument goes, we can find its quality as language by decomposing the iconic whole into an underlying structure of components that are both *arbitrary* and *categorical*.

---

languages, and indeed there is a wide range of iconic patterning found in speech. However, even in languages that feature ideophones prominently, their scope of application appears to be very contained.

2.   From George Sibscota's "The Deaf and Dumb Man's Discourse" (1670):

But those very significations of things, which Mutes make use of, proceed not from nature, but from their own institution no more, than our speech; Therefore they attain unto them by Study and exercise.

Although however most of them do shadow some outward manner, of the things which they aim at. As when they close one hand, and move it up towards the Nostrils, thereby they signifie a Flower. Now the significations of those Mutes (which is as it were their Speech) are not like the Languages which vary among several Nations, nor are so absolutely different.

3.   This book is indebted, in particular, to the phonological research of Wendy Sandler (1989, 2008) and Diane Brentari (1998, 2008), the sociolinguistic histories of Anne Senghas (2004), and the grammatical theory of Scott Liddell (2003).

Witness the sudden and unintended celebrity of Lydia Callis, former New York City mayor Michael Bloomberg's American Sign Language interpreter. Callis became a minor sensation on Twitter and Facebook in the October 2012 run-up to Hurricane Sandy. What made Callis famous—and what infuriated many of her interpreter colleagues—was just how *different* her signing was from the mayor's speaking. In contrast to Bloomberg's torpid and dour delivery of safety tips for storm conditions, Callis's rendering of his words in sign was celebrated as "evocative" and "full of life." Videos of her press conference circulated widely on social media, where enthusiastic nonsigners embraced the possibility that an unlearned language might somehow be more communicatively effective than a politician's drab English. They called her signing "clear," "powerful," and "understandable," and they were joined by none less than Jon Stewart, who characterized her work as "an Alvin Ailey sign language recital" (*The Daily Show*, Oct. 31, 2013). This in turn was met with strident objections by many in the linguistics community, who argued that Callis's apparent evocativeness—especially her facial expressions—was actually an expression of *grammar*. In this statement, what they sought to reveal to public notice was an underlying logic of arbitrary rules, driving the shape and realization of signs much like noun case in Latin or vowel harmony in Turkish (Okrent 2012). The fact that much of Callis's signing *looked like* what it was intended to mean was cast as incidental or, at most, a relic of etymologies long since ossified. Politics of recognition aside, the debate turns on a very important question: To be linguistic, must sign language also be arbitrary?

To many in the West, at least, the answer appears to be *yes*. Though the particulars of dual patterning have always been controversial, the larger principle of form through the composition of arbitrary parts has remained largely unchallenged in linguistics. According to this framework, language works as a basis of intersubjectivity because we all know it, individually. Problems of intelligibility, then, are at most a fait accompli of a more general fact of formal competency. This principle drives and substantiates the arbitrariness of code, and it appears to be so basic to Euro-American ideologies of language that even the possibility of nonarbitrariness occurs often enough to put the question of language itself at stake. The spirit of this dilemma was best exemplified years ago by linguists Edward Klima and Ursula Bellugi, whose seminal book on ASL, *Signs of Language*, set the program of research on signing for decades. In a particularly reflective methodological section, they state:

When we analyze a typical conversation or narrative among deaf signers, we find that nearly all of the manual gestures that are made are ASL signs. Actual ASL signs are a rich set of conventional symbols that conform to a specific set of systematic formation constraints that distinguish American Sign Language from other sign languages and from gestures in general. . . . We shall call a certain set of nonsigning gestures that occur in deaf communication "mimetic representation." The amount of such mimetic representation varies, of course, from individual to individual and from situation to situation. It is significant that in deaf communication, the sign-symbolic (i.e., the "linguistic") and the mimetic are in the same channel. Deaf signers, however, have a very strong sense of the difference between the extremes: between what counts as an ASL sign and what is clearly pantomime. (Klima and Bellugi 1979, 515)

Given the range and rhythm of deaf communicative practices described in the earlier chapters of this book, it should be no surprise that I reject on broad methodological grounds Klima and Bellugi's impulse to distill *language* from *mimetic representation*.[4] Nevertheless, my aim here is not to settle any debates about the relationship between signing and gesture. Rather, in this chapter, I intend to use Klima and Bellugi's very emblematic framework as a starting point to elaborate deaf theories of language in contemporary Kathmandu. The activists I knew had strong intuitions about the differences between good language and bad, and to these intuitions they attached very particular hopes for what NSL might be. Though their analysis can at times appear to map Klima and Bellugi's distinction between the iconic and the arbitrary, I think it is a mistake to fall into these categories too easily. Instead, deaf ways of imagining language in Nepal are built on very different ontological insights.

. . . THE LONG AND THE SHORT

In its mature form, NSL is a recent phenomenon, though how far back its roots go is really anyone's guess. Nevertheless, it is reasonable to say that the

---

4.   To this end, I join a growing body of work that has sought to reevaluate the distinction between language and gesture from a more specifically linguistic perspective (see especially Taub 2001; Quinto-Pozos 2007, 2010; and Cormier et al. 2012).

conditions of its possibility as a public language first came together only in the late 1960s when Nepal's first deaf institutions provided contexts in which the deaf could interact with each other in substantial and sustained ways. Though we know very little about NSL's earliest structure, the language was undoubtedly first informed by a process that unified and extended a number of idiosyncratic "home sign" systems (Hoffmann-Dilloway 2011; Brentari et al. 2012). These antecedents to NSL, built from necessity in domestic spaces, were generally confined to a single family, a single generation, and, more often than not, a very rudimentary basis of content. Since then, of course, NSL has emerged as a fully capable language, though the mechanism and character of this process of transformation are—I think it is fair to say—still very poorly understood. As one would expect, each branch of the academy has its own explanations based on its own theoretical commitments. The cognitive psychologists have their generative brains, the sociobiologists have their exigencies of fitness, and the anthropologists have their semiotic manifest destiny. Beneath all this apparent disputation, however, is a single relatively consistent narrative: if you put a bunch of deaf people together, language quickly shows up (Senghas 2004, 2005; Sandler et al. 2011).

It is the general position of Nepali deaf activism that this line of reasoning demonstrates a deeply superstitious understanding of the world. The idea that language could come from nonlanguage, they say, is profoundly unscientific—magical, even—like believing that life can emerge from broth and vital ether in a world before Pasteur. According to deaf Nepal's reckoning—or, at least, in its most colorful rendition of the tale—the potentialities of sign language did not emerge on their own but were instead *given* to Nepalis by a bunch of Italian deaf hippies sometime in the 1970s. The telling of this story usually features a small group of Nepali deaf teenagers, typically including Raghav Bir Joshi and several other well-known community leaders. As the story goes, they were sitting beneath the national martyrs' monument near New Road, idly chatting and passing the time. Suddenly, from across the parade ground, they saw several foreign tourists, shrouded in oily smoke and talking furiously with their hands. In the most extreme versions of this story, the encounter lasted only a moment: they met eyes, exchanged greetings, and then went their separate ways. Though many (including Mr. Joshi) are quick to point out that the interaction was actually quite a bit more substantial than this, enthusiastic retellers have boiled the story down to its barest elements: (1) half-baked Johnny Appleseed (2) gave language to deaf Nepal (3) under a national martyrs' monument. As far as creation myths go, Lévi-Strauss would have been proud. According to this account, language wasn't generated but rather transferred, and what is most conspicuous is how much effort goes into making the particularities of that transfer utterly irrelevant to the basis of contact that made it possible. With every subsequent retelling, the meeting gets more brief, the hippies get more stoned, and the transformation gets more transcendent.[5]

My friends in the deaf activist world are not being naïve here. They of course recognize that, even in the decades before the Italians showed up, they were engaged in complexly organized communicative practices of some sort or another and, moreover, that their language continues to change over time. When I asked what it was that they were speaking before meeting the Italians, however, their response was always uncharacteristically terse: "short." My requests for elaboration were met with friendly impatience. "Short" was an obvious synonym of casual, bad, empty, or (in an idiom particularly salient in Nepal) underdeveloped (cf. Bista 1991). It just meant "what we had before that is worse than what we have now." In these accounts, the character of "short" language is both underspecified and ideologically charged, linked more to the kinds of people who use "short" language than to any particular set of linguistic structures. To draw from a litany of descriptions offered by deaf activists over several years of fieldwork, users of "short" are "uneducated," "without sense and reason," "natural," "unmodern," and "mentally handicapped." They are, in other words, precisely what the hearing tend to think the deaf are.

Over the past ten years, a constellation of deaf political, social, and welfare organizations has asserted effective claim over better and worse forms of signing. Though they are diverse in form and purpose, these organizations have demonstrated a consistent and clear intention to promulgate NSL as a very particular kind of sign language used by a very particular kind of speaker. Much of what I described in chapter 3 would fall under the category "short," just as it would be described as "gesture" in the American linguistics literature. Critically, however, "short" and "gesture" should not be understood as isomorphic terms. In this section, I will suggest that explicitly institutional anxieties about "short"

---

5. Since my primary fieldwork ended, several of the Italians have actually returned to Kathmandu to visit. This has significantly reanchored the narrative described here to historical events. Nevertheless, I present the idealized version of the story because the direction of its drift is more telling than the actual particulars.

language—rather than tensions between iconic gesture and arbitrary sign—configure and motivate the deaf activist project in its ambitions to disseminate NSL throughout the country.

The dialog that serves as the primary ethnographic data for this section took place in 2011 at the "Older and Vulnerable Deaf Persons' Project" in Kathmandu. This project is administered by KAD with financial support from DeafWay UK. It aims to provide education and socialization opportunities to economically marginal deaf adults, chiefly through a generous day program featuring skills training and meal provisions. Our cast has two primary actors: the first, an elderly deaf man, is a native signer. Though he has not participated much in the language standardization projects put forward by the institutions speaking on behalf of Nepali deaf activism, he has been a part of the broader community for his entire life. Most importantly, he is the quintessence of "short" signers.[6] Consequently, and despite having used sign to communicate effectively with both the deaf and the hearing for decades, he has been selected by this program for a course in basic sign language. I've called him Mr. Short. His teacher, whom I've called Ms. Long, is a young hearing woman who has herself recently undergone a pedagogically similar four-month course at KAD. It is important to note that she is in her position only temporarily. She is acting as a substitute for the regular teacher, who is deaf and who has been absent for several weeks. As a consequence, Ms. Long does not know Mr. Short very well.

The interaction described here was fast-paced, unfolding over just a few minutes in real time. The teacher, Ms. Long, has written the word "cow" in Nepali's Devanagari script on the classroom's whiteboard. She is trying to prompt her charge of signers to place their thumbs on their forehead with their index fingers extended outward. This is the sign for "cow" in the official NSL dictionary (figure 12). Mr. Short comes to produce this form only after considerable miscommunication and, as would be unambiguous to an NSL-savvy viewer, the eight failed attempts that came before his ultimately successful one exemplify "short" language practices. As I will explain, they were deemed to fail for exactly this reason. The overarching structure of the interaction is nine adjacency pairs (alternating "turns" in the interaction), each of which is composed by an attempt at elicitation by Ms. Long and an unsuccessful response from Mr. Short. At two moments, Mr. Short recalibrates his interpretation of

---

6.   For a variationist account of NSL as it is used by older signers, see Khanal (2013).

Ms. Long's expectations, and I have used these two shifts to break the text into three parts:[7]

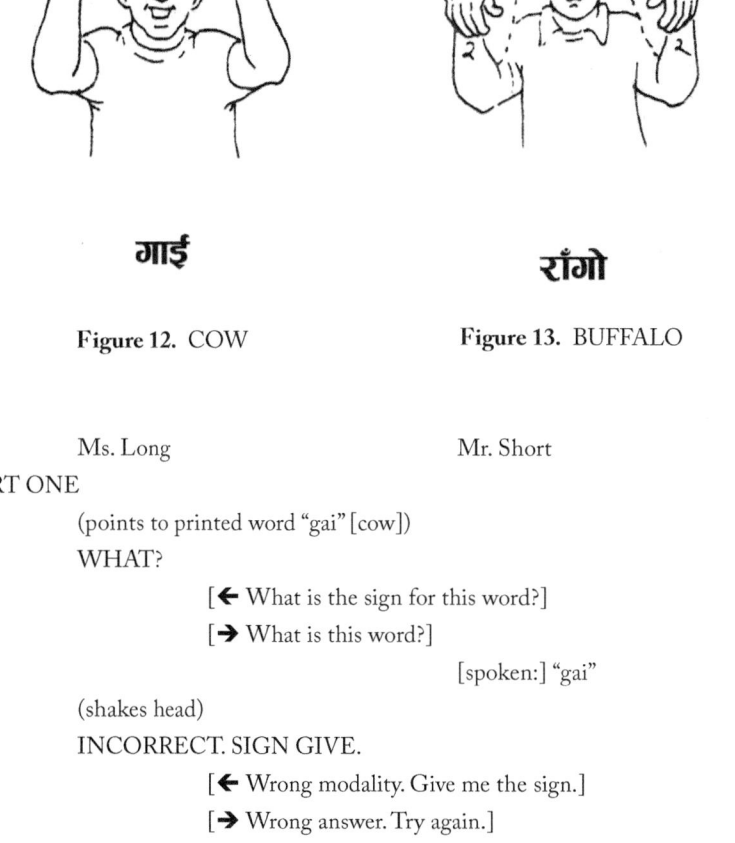

गाई   राँगो

Figure 12. COW   **Figure 13.** BUFFALO

	Ms. Long	Mr. Short

PART ONE

1a)   (points to printed word "gai" [cow])
           WHAT?
                         [← What is the sign for this word?]
                         [→ What is this word?]
1b)   [spoken:] "gai"
2a)   (shakes head)
           INCORRECT. SIGN GIVE.
                         [← Wrong modality. Give me the sign.]
                         [→ Wrong answer. Try again.]
2b)   [spoken, emphatically:] "gai"

---

7.   Conventions of glossing: CAPITALIZED WORDS are glosses for standardized lexical entries from the NSL dictionary. When two or more English words are required to indicate a single conventional sign, THEY_ARE_JOINED by an underscore. (words in parentheses) are descriptions of nonstandardized productions in the signing channel. [words in brackets] are contextual explanations and interpretations of speaker intention. [← left arrows] indicate speaker intention. [→ right arrows] indicate apparent interpretation.

3a)   SIGN GIVE

                 [← Give me the sign.]

                 [→ I don't understand.]

3b)   (points to picture of a cow)

PART TWO

4a)   Student: SEE SEE SEE

                 [← She wants to see the sign.]

                 [→ She wants to see the sign.]

4b)   (curved horns) [= cow]

5a)   (points to picture of buffalo)

       BUFFALO INCORRECT. COW

                 [← That's the sign for "buffalo." I want "cow."]

                 [→ I'm not understanding you.]

5b)   AGREE.

                                (curved horns, give tika,

                                lumbering gait . . .)

PART THREE

6a)   WORD WORD WORD WORD WORD TOO_MUCH. COW.

                 [← This is too many words. Just COW.]

                 [→ This is too many words. Just "cow."]

6b)   (index fingers at back of head)

                                [= cow]

7a)   COW.

                 [← Your sign is incorrect.]

                 [→ Your sign doesn't look like a cow.]

7b)   [emphasizing back and hooked

                                shape:]

                                (index fingers at back of head)

8a)   COW.

                 [← No, this is correct.]

                 [→ No, this is better.]

8b)   [turns to audience]

                                (index fingers at back of head)

                                [= isn't this a better cow?]

9a)   [physically moves hands to desired sign]

9b)   COW! [laughing]

To begin, Ms Long summons Mr. Short to the front of the classroom. Once he is there, she points to the word "गाई" on her whiteboard. This is the Nepali word for cow (1a). Mr. Short, who (like many deaf people) has learned how to speak to some extent, responds in reasonably clear spoken Nepali: "*gāi*," or "cow" (1b).

"INCORRECT," Ms. Long tells him. She was looking for a signed rather than spoken token, and so she prompts Mr. Short to try again. In order to clarify her intentions, she adds a phrase "SIGN GIVE" (2a). For her, this is an obvious and explicit attempt to switch the conversation over to a signing channel. Mr. Short, however, does not perceive these particularities in her request, and so instead he concludes that the problem was that his vocalization wasn't clear enough. The logical course of this misunderstanding is important. In colloquial NSL, the lexical form SIGN can be used (with the correct rapid-fire prosody and puzzled facial expression) to mean something like "I don't understand what you're talking about. Try again differently." It is a request for clarification, but not one that necessarily demands a signing channel in preference to any other. This use of "SIGN" to mean more than just signing is not particularly unusual. After all, deaf voice is constituted through a wide range of modalities, and though signing is the most important it remains only one among many. As far as Mr. Short is concerned, speech is a perfectly appropriate response to SIGN GIVE, because SIGN itself refers in the absence of further specificity to all forms of communication. For the deaf, including verbal speech under the rubric of "sign" is no stranger than when the hearing describe conversations over email as a kind of "talking." These nuances of deaf experience are lost on Ms. Long, however, who encounters SIGN more markedly as obviously and inherently contrastive against everything spoken. So, miscalibrated to these intentions, Mr. Short repeats himself, this time with more enthusiasm: "*gāi!*" (2b). Again, Ms. Long blocks Mr. Short, and asks him to SIGN (3a). Visibly frustrated, Mr. Short walks over to a classroom wall covered with pictures, finds a photo of a cow, and points at it (3b).

At this moment, another student intervenes in the miscommunication to explain—accurately and more intelligibly—what Ms. Long actually wants (4a). She wants Mr. Short not only to reference "cow," but moreover to do it *specifically* with manual signs. This intervention came none too soon, because by this point Mr. Short had started to imply (only somewhat facetiously, I think) that he might go down to the street to haul a living cow up the two flights of stairs into the classroom. When a hearing person isn't understanding you, a good signer knows not to shift up the hierarchy of intelligible reference to conventional forms but rather down to material props. As previously described, these instincts are fundamental to effective signing in Nepal. But it is no accident that Ms. Long, the only hearing person present aside from myself and the only nonnative signer then employed by KAD, was selected to teach this class. Her limited experience with sign language outside of classroom settings has left her unable to effectively negotiate the metalinguistic aspects of this exchange, at least in terms that would feel coherent to the more nuanced functional intuitions of Mr. Short. Instead, she pursues a context of exchange oriented narrowly and explicitly around the normative sign forms listed in the NSL dictionary. This is, however, a strikingly alien place for Mr. Short to be. Indeed, against the dictionary's inventory of words, Mr. Short has spent his entire life honing a capacity to be denotationally effective to the hearing by whatever means are most ready at his disposal. He understands that he is at this moment failing at that goal, but he doesn't understand why.

The missing piece here is simple: Mr. Short does not know that he has been invited to this classroom today to learn sign language, and outside of that particular contextual framing, it doesn't seem particularly sensible for him to respond to Ms. Long (a hearing woman) in a signed channel. He believes, instead, that he is here to learn to read, and so he understands the purpose of his task to be the effective interpretation of the marks drawn in pen on the whiteboard. Having successfully read and understood the word to himself, the channel of response in which his answer is delivered to Ms. Long seems to him entirely secondary to whether or not his answer is correct. He thus chose to speak "cow" rather than sign "COW" because doing so seemed to be the most effective way to participate in this interaction with the hearing Ms. Long.

Now that the matter of signing versus speaking has been clarified, however, Mr. Short is ready to move forward. He responds to the prompt once again by placing his palms against his forehead and moving them forward in the outline of curved horns (4b). This structures another major miscommunication. Ms. Long, in her four-month sign language course, was taught the 2,202 signs in the official *Nepali Sign Language Dictionary* and virtually nothing else. In that dictionary, the particular structure of motion that Mr. Short produced is identical to the official sign for "buffalo" (figure 13) but wholly different from the sign for "cow." Mr. Short, who has spent most of his life successfully signing outside this standard, has no idea of this fact. Though he could no doubt distinguish both cognitively and communicatively between cows and buffalos if the need arose, that difference does not obtain for him over strict lexical distinctions. He is not, in other words, invested in the problem of denotation primarily as a question of names. Rather, his strategy here is to reference cows by reproducing a perceptually salient feature of them—their curved horns, which he selected for this context on the basis of his intuitions about what will be visually salient to Ms. Long about cows and cowhood. In the present context where the goal is communicative efficacy and where a distinction between cows and buffalos does not seem particularly relevant, Mr. Short would find the possibility that he could somehow reference buffalos *accidentally* to be perplexing. He believes that—in this here-and-now—curved horns should be enough on their own to indicate that he has successfully interpreted the markings on the whiteboard. Ms. Long, who contends that this is simply incorrect, continues to object.

But Mr. Short does not interpret Ms. Long's continuing objections (5a) in these terms. In all reality, he likely has no idea that such a thing as an NSL dictionary even exists. Instead, he takes his teacher's protestations to be about the clarity of his iconic mappings. To this end, he understands her juxtaposition of two different representations of curved horns as a request for further elaboration, so he goes on to elect other contextually salient traits of cows: they receive *tika* markings on their foreheads from religious practitioners, they eat grass, they lumber down the road right outside here with a heavy gait, they cause traffic jams, and so on (5b). By the conventions of signed referential practice, his rhythm and pacing indicate that he will keep going with these elaborations until Ms. Long signals that his meaning has been made sufficiently clear. Of course, no amount of elaboration will ever be enough because Ms. Long is waiting for a specific, arbitrary lexical convention. He wants to be effective, but she wants him to be right.

Eventually, Ms. Long tells Mr. Short that he is being too wordy (6a), and he again recalibrates his expectations. He produces a new sign for "cow"—concise this time—with hooked index fingers at the back of his head (6b). This is, of course, still not the sign Ms. Long is looking for (7a). She chastises him and offers her correct answer yet again. Mr. Short has by now decided that the entire situation is hilarious. Though he maintains a semblance of bemused ignorance about the cause of his struggles, the exasperated pleas of his classmates ("You know the sign she wants, get on with it!") suggest that he might by this point just be egging her on. Whatever the case may be, he finds her sign inferior to his own. He doesn't like the fact that she places her horns at the front of her head rather than farther back, and he doesn't like the sharp angle of their curve (7b).

His objections are irrelevant, however, because she holds fundamental the idea that words are conventions and thus are not subject to evaluation by individuals in real-time discourse. In her NSL but critically not in his, there are no better signs or worse signs, only correct ones and incorrect ones. On this matter, both sides are entrenched and both sides have begun to repeat themselves. After her third failure at elicitation, Ms. Long finally acknowledges the impasse (8a + 8b). Defeated (though enjoying herself nevertheless), she walks over to Mr. Short, takes his hands, and physically repositions them in the shape and location she has been seeking (9a). Mr. Short turns to his audience of classmates and presents Ms. Long's sign—thumbs at forehead, sharply angled—saturated with hammy enthusiasm (9b).

A prominent member of the Nepali Sign Language National Development Committee witnessed this interaction with me. I later asked her for her assessment of Mr. Short, and her response was familiar: "He's uneducated. I don't understand his talk. How am I supposed to understand that? It's empty. Forget it." She had no trouble recounting the content of the conversation, however, so the parts of his talk that she cannot understand are clearly not to be fixed on any question of meaning per se. There is, rather, something else unintelligible to her about him. Mr. Short was similarly critical of his experience, describing his teacher thus:

> Her signing is terrible. How am I supposed to understand any of it? . . . If I went up to a shopkeeper and asked for some cow milk saying cow like how she wants [with sharply angled horns] . . . what is this, a deer? Deer milk? And when someone doesn't understand, she just keeps doing the same thing over and over again.

The easy analysis to be made here begins in terms of disparities of power. Mr. Short and Ms. Long are representatives of opposed understandings of what NSL is and how it ought to be, and they stand differently in their evaluations of good signing and bad. They are not, however, the same kinds of people. It is no surprise that Ms. Long, with her institutional backing and political clout, ultimately wins. Likewise, it is no surprise that Mr. Short and his language come to be emblematic of everything ignorant and underdeveloped. But what I wish to draw attention to in this exchange goes well beyond mere symbolic associations between kinds of language and kinds of people. More broadly, formal elicitation in this classroom setting casts speech as a function of preferred correspondences between words and things. Though the source of these preferences is unambiguously the NSL dictionary, understanding what invests that dictionary with this power requires quite a bit more work. It is tempting to read these standardization narratives as institutional attempts to draw a line between arbitrary language and iconic gesture, but I believe that this interpretation is a mistake, placing the cart before the proverbial cow and/or buffalo. To reframe these questions from a deaf perspective instead, we must better understand what distinguishes the *long* and the *short*. For this, we must trace the gap between what is intelligible to hearing linguists and to deaf activists in the presence of words.

DEAF LINGUISTIC THEORY

If signers intuitively discern the difference between gesture and language, as Klima and Bellugi suggest, we would expect language standardization projects to privilege this distinction above all else. In deaf Nepal, however, neither the signers nor the nonsigners I knew were very interested in these categories. Here, the problem of iconic forms and arbitrary forms emerges from a very different set of problems than those anticipated by the Euro-American tradition. Consequently, to understand the limits of *short* and the merits of *long* language, we must begin instead with a more local inventory of assumptions about how it is that languages exist in the first place.

For starters, deaf people really *like* the parts of NSL that the hearing most often fail to see as linguistic. They like being able to communicate effectively even in the absence of a shared formal code, and the fact that they can do so (they constantly reminded me) should make it obvious to everyone that NSL is just *better* than hearing languages in some fundamental ways. This appeal to the value of transparency is so fundamental to deaf ambitions for their language that it shapes even how its most explicitly arbitrary conventions are organized. At one meeting of the NSL National Development Committee, for example, I witnessed a heated dispute over what would ultimately become the official sign for "jet ski." As far as conventionalizing impulses go, the fact that this question could even come up goes to demonstrate just how boundlessly expansive the aspirations of standardization can be. Nepal is a land-locked country with few lakes, deep poverty, and a social topology that makes recreational water sports an unlikely priority for deaf people. Nevertheless, as early work began on an expanded NSL dictionary, everyone agreed that having a sign for jet ski was important. What was also important, they agreed, was that the sign for jet ski capture something fundamental about jet skis themselves. Coming to a consensus about what exactly that meant, however, was more controversial. Several signs were proposed, and each in turn was rebuked for not evoking the *feel* of jet skis vividly enough. As these debates fractured the committee's membership into a dozen or more contentious sides, everyone accused everyone else of not understanding how jet skis *seem* to others. On this point, none of them were wrong. Some signs looked more like whales, it was observed, while others failed to convey that jet skis are in fact quite a bit smaller than speedboats. There was significant discussion about whether the vertical plume of water that some had seen following jet skis on TV was an essential part of their visual form. Far from seeking to escape iconically driven signing, in these debates the core institutions of the NSL standardization project vehemently embraced it (see also Hoffmann 2008; Hoffmann-Dilloway 2011). But if the purpose of a standardization project is to align language to a standardized set of forms, why does iconic transparency matter? If the task of denotation is already sufficiently advanced by a shared knowledge of convention, what does iconicity *do*?

According to a young and famously ambitious deaf teacher whom I'll call Kriti, iconicity is important to NSL because it makes the language *EASY*. The sign being glossed here as "easy" is especially evocative: an index finger points at the temple (indicating thought), followed by a snap and a quick twist of the wrist (indicating speed) (figure 14). When signing is at its best, she explained, it should be both fast and direct, able to move into the minds of others with as little friction as possible. By keeping the meaning of NSL's vocabulary clear, she hoped that the language would be quicker to teach to the deaf and more effective to use with the hearing. Though Kriti is uniquely articulate as an advocate for her language, I heard these same sentiments expressed countless times by many other deaf activists at standardization meetings, teacher trainings, and political assemblies. On Kriti's last point, however, I pushed back. I argued that "better" isn't usually at stake in questions of linguistic form, and I asked why these characteristics are so important for signed languages but not spoken ones. She answered, rather more sharply than had previously been her tone: "Good words are not necessary for them. Hearing people all live together. They don't learn their language in a classroom. They don't have to ask *why* this means that. It doesn't matter for them. The meaning is just there on its own."

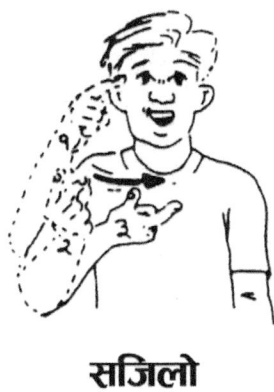

सजिलो

Figure 14. EASY

In this statement, Kriti was highlighting for me a dimension of deaf experience that had been brought to my attention so many times before: namely, the hearing don't have to think about *how* language works, but the deaf—constantly—do; these asymmetries of experience are manifest in the very different extents to which language is intelligible in context to them. Where the hearing look at words and see meaning, the deaf see instead diverse architectures of correspondence with their vast social histories intact. In light of these differences, it is especially noteworthy that Kriti talks about NSL in this way to include even the signing that she does with *nonsigners*. This is unusual. The hearing don't generally know NSL, of course, but nevertheless it would seem that NSL is a kind of thing capable of being projected upon them. By including the hearing in this way as first-order participants in signing's community of relevance, the deaf make a remarkable choice. They stipulate their language as a social fact with very unexpected boundaries, and they invite its comparison to more familiar spoken languages in terms that demand deep shifts of attention. Though it is evident from Kriti's words and actions that she is personally invested in the idea of a linguistic standard for NSL, the question of *what* exactly she hopes will be standardized remains conspicuously unclear.

At this point in our conversation, another teacher watching intervened. I recognized the man but didn't know his name. I'd seen him at many teachers' training events in the past, but he was quiet and I'm not sure I'd ever seen him speak. Now, however, he turned to challenge me directly: "You want to make NSL's vocabulary fixed [lit. "lined up in a row"]. You want to make it bigger, so all of the deaf people can know the same words and be together that way. That's good, but it's only half."

He stopped there and waited for me to respond. As far as I could remember, I had never actually advocated for an expanded anything to him or anyone else, but the rhetorical dynamic at play in his statement was one I encountered often. In the absence of a hearing public to which the deaf can easily speak, I often found myself mobilized as a proxy for untenable hearing mindsets. I had, in this adopted role, misunderstood the goals of NSL's standardization by seeing it in terms too familiar to the hearing. I had, specifically, expected it to be motivated by the same sociopolitical ambitions of identity, ethnicity, separation, and autonomy that carry forward Nepal's many variously construed linguistic nationalisms. What the deaf aspire to, however, is something very different, and I needed to understand that difference if I wished to understand the deaf. Dutifully, I responded, "So what's the other half?" He explained, "The other half is how to make a line of connection between the deaf and the hearing. The deaf are over here and the hearing are over there, but there is a wall between them. When signs are clear, they open that wall." The "wall" in this phrasing was made using the flats of two hands to create a barrier between the left side of the signing space and the right, separating where the deaf and the hearing had been previously established as spatial pronouns. The sign CLEAR, which is generally made by moving two flat hands apart from each other in a lateral motion (figure 15), was being inflected here to make it mimic the motion of a gate in that wall. Clarity, in other words, opens up the world. When deaf Nepal hopes for a standardized language, what it hopes for is not merely uptake and consistency for its scattered community but, moreover, a corpus of perfect signs that can pass through the many barriers that enclose deaf places.

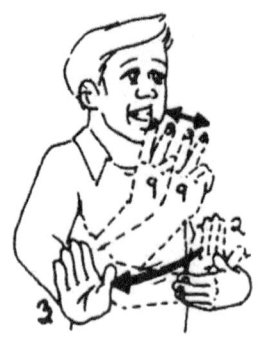

स्पष्ट

Figure 15. CLEAR

In this question of perfection, deaf activists reveal their very complex relationship to broader theories of language in the region. Though Euro-American traditions have for millennia tended to subsume language function under the banner of cognition and denotative reference, South Asian thought has instead concerned itself chiefly with the *instrumental* properties of sound (see below, and especially Wilke and Moebus 2011). This is a subtly implicated difference, rooted in a long history of speculation about the nature of language generally and the language of the Hindu Vedas specifically. The Vedas, in their most tangible sense, are a collection of religious texts. They are extremely old and often quite cryptic, and scholars have been commenting on both this age and this opacity for nearly three thousand years now (especially as regards the nature and purpose of their language; see Kelly 1996). The importance of this scholarship to South Asian philosophy cannot be easily overstated. In a very literal sense, the Vedas are the Ur-thing against which all other things are said to be. Even and especially for those who reject their scriptural authority (Buddhists, for example), the ontology of Vedic language has provided a starting point for an extremely diverse history of thought. For much of the region's past and present, making a claim about the Vedas has been synonymous with making a claim about the nature of reality itself.

What is important to know about the Vedas is that they exist to orthodox interpretations not chiefly as communicative texts but rather as direct, effective action. To recite the Vedas is not to *express* something but rather to *do* something (Smith 1986; Patton 2011). This ascription to efficacy is not merely a theory of speech acts or magic, however. Quite to the contrary, what is most important about the Vedas is precisely their total exemption from any kind of event-structure (see, e.g., Paudel 2010). It is often said that the Vedas are "timeless," but even that claim does not go far enough because their transcendence is not merely temporal. The Vedas are not of human provenance, but neither are they divine revelations in any agentive sense. Rather, they are a thing much more basic. They are, quite concretely, a property of the world in exactly the way that audibility is a property of sound.

Though many of Nepal's non-Hindu communities reject the primacy of the Vedas either more or less explicitly, the broader metaphysics of a *true* language emergent from reality itself remain more pervasively intact. Across the diversity of Nepal's interconnected traditions of shamanism, for example, healing is often accomplished by detecting and engaging the autochthonic link between words and things. As Gregory Maskarinec describes in his ethnography of discursive practices among Nepali shamans, "The shaman pounds on his words just like he pounds on his drum, as if to shatter them, testing the elasticity of language, pulling it apart to reveal the most vulnerable parts of the world, where it may be most susceptible to manipulation" (Maskarinec 1995, 242, also 192). What, then, about sign? Would truly *prakṛtik* signs, formed within the spaces of anti-consciousness described in chapter 3, have the same powers of direct efficacy? And what about the institutionally sanctioned transparency under constant pursuit by the NSL National Development Committee? When I asked Kriti these questions, she just rolled her eyes and snorted. These were garbage super-stitions, she said, taken seriously only by ignorant villagers. She asked me if I believed in *jhānkris* (shamans), and—caught off guard—I muttered something anthropological about the social viability of diverse belief systems. At this, she visibly grimaced, and told me that I should decide for myself what I believe.

A few weeks later, however, Kriti raised the issue again, this time more neutrally. We were waiting at KAD with a half dozen others to meet a deaf tourist on her way through town, and we were passing the time in aimless conversation. At a lull in our talk, Kriti repeated my question for others to hear: "Just as a thought experiment [lit. 'thought spinning from the head and going far away']," she said, "could *jhānkris* use sign language?" Most just shrugged their shoulders, but one man in his early twenties replied after taking several moments to think:

> When the *jhānkri* speaks and plays the drum, the sound penetrates the sick person's body. It goes inside and . . . well, I don't know if it actually works. I don't think it does. But signs are made from our hands, and the light bounces off of them. I don't think it can penetrate in the same way. Anyway, the diseases that *jhānkris* cure are hearing diseases. If there were deaf diseases, maybe a signing *jhānkri* could cure them, but I don't think there are any.

This was the first time I'd ever heard mention of "deaf diseases," though nobody else in the room took exception to the phrase. When I pushed for elaboration, however, the young man became visibly frustrated: "There are no deaf diseas-es, so it doesn't mean anything." I asked whether something like cancer was a deaf or hearing disease, and without hesitation he replied, "It's both. That's why *jhānkris* can't cure it. They can only cure hearing diseases." When I asked what constituted hearing diseases, he once again shrugged: "You know. All the things that hospitals can't cure but *jhānkris* can."

In these moments, we begin to see the stakes of sound's very material presence. The deaf and the hearing occupy very different causal domains, but, for the purposes of linguistic efficacy, these domains are not merely *separate*. Indeed, as a thought experiment of my own, I approached several practicing Brahmin priests about the possibility of translating some of the Vedas' more famous hymns into NSL. Though they praised the ambitions they assumed I had to offer spiritual opportunities to deaf people, they all agreed that my project was utterly unrealizable. The problem was simple: the Vedas are a collection of mantras, each of which is an elaboration of the *pranava* mantra, "Aum." Though mantras are often characterized in casual terms as prayers or meditations, this ascription to purpose ultimately misses the point entirely (cf. Yelle 2003). Mantras are, much more basically, sounds. Though we might introspect upon them, identify their components, and translate them into other forms of representation, our capacity to do so is ultimately incidental to the fact that they exist—primally and exclusively—as the basic detectable presence of the sounds that they are. Though the implications of the Vedas for the world are indeed vast, their existence is in total neither more nor less than their very specific acoustic properties. As a consequence, my consultants explained, translating the Vedas into Nepali or English is already bad enough, but at least there the efficacy of sound remains in some form. NSL, as a silent language, was just a total nonstarter. With kindly hopes of salvaging my project, however, several noted the existence of *mudras*, ritual gestures that often accompany Vedic recitation, and a few suggested enthusiastically that the deaf might already have deep predilections in this direction. But, ultimately, I needed to understand that mudras and mantras are very different things, and there was to be no question of translating one into the other. Doing so, in the words of one priest, "would be like trying to play cricket with the beam of a flashlight."

Though these priests offered many statements of sympathy for the deaf and their plight, with varying amounts of embarrassment they all ultimately admitted that there was very little that they could do to help. In their worlds, the deaf *lacked* something with no possible substitute. In Hindu cosmogony, sound is just no ordinary thing. Rather, it is the dimension of reality most consubstantial with the fact of creation itself. The Vedic sacrifice—organized around the careful recitation of mantras—is designed as an expressly acoustic experience, imitating in this regard the primordial sacrifice that first established the distinctive contours of our shared reality. What the deaf reportedly lack in their nonperception of sound is not just these rituals, however, but something far more fundamental. As the priests explained to me, when the sensible world came to be, substance and consciousness arose from *brahman*, a unity so basic that even questions of existence or nonexistence are subsequent to it (Matilal 1998, 21). Against this background state, *particularity* always comes as a disruption, a separation accounted for against that which is prior to it (Coward 1990, 60). Notably, however, the disruption caused by this emergence of particularity always bears traces in distinctly kinetic terms. It refracts through the world and through consciousness to yield countless manifestations, each of which is undergirded by an essential *audible* vibration (Beck 1993, 121). As a consequence, the experience of sound is the experience of these vibrations in their most basic manifestation, and acts of careful mindfulness can teach us to hear relatively more of them. This is why, for example, the mantras of the Vedas are described not as words discovered, received, or remembered like most other religious texts but rather as something "heard" (*smṛti*), detected in the world itself by sages long dead as their echoes reverberated across time from the fact of creation. Thus, when Vedic commentators suggest that the creation of the universe is identical to the sound *Aum*, the claim is not meant as a flight of metaphor. *Aum* is the extent of the world in all its particularity, and all other mantras are proximal elaborations on it. Acts of verbal recitation are thus not merely a reference to but rather a direct enactment of the everything as it exists (Yelle 2003, 27). In these terms, sound is the substance of everything more specific than totality. Everything that *is* is also sound (Ganeri 1999, vii).

It should go without saying that the implications for the deaf of a reality made out of sound are vast. According to these ways of thinking, all phenomenologically accessible presences are correctly understood as sites of engagement not with the world but rather with the echoes made particular of an unparticular primacy of being (Wilke and Moebus 2011). What we might call "reality" is thus equally present in all things and all perceptions, ready to be heard by those who can. What makes the Vedas specifically untranslatable into sign is the same thing that makes them unique: their state of relative preservation in specifically acoustic terms. They are the only remnants still intact from the moment of creation itself, free from the distortion of time and misperception (Deshpande 1993; Pollock 2006, 27). Everything else has just been around too long to remain true, distorted over time by the systematic patterns of misperception that accumulate in social institutions. Our shared reality, according to this reckoning, has become faded, like photocopies of photocopies of photocopies. Recitation of the Vedas seeks harmonization—in a literal acoustic sense—with the fact of *brahman* as universal. Through proper and correct speech, it is thus possible to realize one's coidentity with totality. To these ends, the collection of mantra sounds that constitutes the Vedas is not merely an account of *brahman*. It is not a representation of *brahman*. It is not a cause or invocation of *brahman*. It *is brahman*, or at least the closest thing to it that remains knowable. Everything else is an echo, slowly degrading over time.

To appreciate the difference between *short* and *long* signing, this question of echoes is paramount. In deaf contexts, echoes are at risk whenever signs are taken from one place or time to another, where imperfect citation can infest them with irrecoverable deviations from an original form. I witnessed this concern across many different contexts but most vividly when I sat in for several months on a class being taught by Kriti at KAD designed to train future interpreters. I had attended a similar course myself several years earlier, but in the interim her pedagogy had taken on a much more formal structure. At the beginning of each hour-long session, Kriti would instruct her class to turn to a specific chapter in the NSL dictionary. Then, keeping rhythm with a stick she tapped on the floor, she would direct her students to read off each of the signs on the page, column by column and row by row. She had seen this technique, she said, in the monastery schools in Boudha, though she wondered how the teachers there could hear individuals amidst the cacophony of voices. With NSL, it was much easier to watch her charges one at a time, which she did vigilantly from the corner of the room. When she observed a sign being produced incorrectly, she would tap her stick twice in quick succession, cueing her students to stop. She would then summon the erring student to the front of the class, where she would ask him or her to recreate the mistake for everyone else to see. If the student tried to make the sign correctly this time, Kriti would interrupt and recreate the malformation herself. The purpose of these drills, it seemed, was not simply to demonstrate correct forms but also to showcase the range of mistakes that might be made. She would use these mistakes as opportunities to expound on how even slightly flawed execution might betray the logic of motivation that the NSL National Development Committee had so meticulously crafted. Keeping one's hands just a bit too far apart when making the sign DOG (figure 16), for example, might confuse someone unfamiliar into thinking that the conversation was about digging, or rabbits, or perhaps even washing a car. Tilting one's head too sharply forward when making the sign WORK (figure 17), meanwhile, might give the impression that deaf people are lazy. In Kriti's class, transparency was always the most important thing, but maintaining transparency in these standardized modalities required very different techniques of attention than those at play in more ad hoc engagements with meaning and form. It required, specifically, a disciplined and precise knowledge of what had been decided at some point in the past by representatives of the deaf community. It *matters* whether jet skis project vertical plumes of water behind them, in this sense, because the decisions made on the basis of these questions are destined to become a permanent part of deaf worlds crafted by NSL's visual ethos.

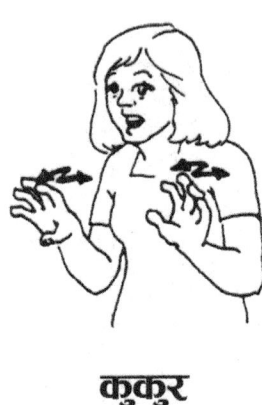

कुकुर

Figure 16. DOG

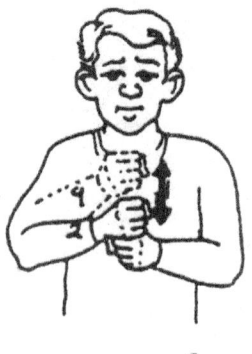

काम गर्नु

Figure 17. WORK

After watching this pattern of instruction unfold for several weeks, I approached Kriti after class one day and asked her if there wasn't perhaps a better way. After all, the interpreters who graduated from these programs tended to be fairly incompetent. They could recite a decent amount of vocabulary, but they had no real sense of how to string a sentence together in the presence of actual deaf people. What about some conversation practice, or even mock scenarios that could simulate what it's like to interpret at community events, at doctors' offices, or at political speeches? Kriti paused, smiled, and asked, "You think this is the same as all Asian education? Too R-O-T-E?" She spelled out this last word in English. I answered that I didn't know about all of Asia, but that I thought her would-be interpreters might benefit from some more realistic kinds of experience. She replied again, this time without hesitation:

> This isn't that. These interpreters, they'll learn all those things later. But now, they need to learn these signs exactly right, because they'll teach these signs to so many other people. If there are mistakes, those mistakes will expand as they go from one person to the next and then to the next and then to the next. The signs will get shorter and shorter and shorter and shorter until there's nothing left.

Short sign, she explained, had two different kinds. There are the signs that people make up themselves, external to the consensus of the deaf community. This, I suspect, is how she would have characterized the various signs for "cow" rejected by Ms. Long in the previous section. The other side of *short*, however, was in her reckoning far more insidious. Even signs built by the deaf community can become abbreviated over time, made simpler by a process of change she dismissed as "LAZY." Maybe someone finds it easier to make the sign for "cow" using only one hand instead of two, or maybe the angle of the horns changes to a more relaxed shape. Maybe eventually they decay to the point where they are no longer recognizable by themselves. These reduced signs remain useful among pockets of friends, perhaps, but they fail utterly to engage the diversity of the deaf community and especially the hearing. Thus, we have two kinds of *short*: one that is too broad and one that is too narrow; one includes nonsigners too completely and the other not at all. The trick for standard NSL is always finding the balance.

According to the linguistic theory of deaf Nepal, the use of language is always an act of *reminding*, a bringing something from the past into the present in order to reinvoke it. Various lower components of structure might be abstracted from these utterances by human minds, but this is always an act of *renvoi*. As a consequence, the basis of form that preserves language and carries it forward from the past to the present is its own particular history of recitation. To this deaf and South Asian formulation, a *sign* should be understood not as a formal object bearing language structure but rather as the causal root—the intention—of an utterance purposely directed at another. In this regard, all signs—iconic, arbitrary, or any various combination thereof—are carved by the demands of what Bhartṛhari calls "mutual expectancy" (ākāṅkṣa) (Bhartṛhari n.d., II.3). People are able to use signs in communication because they can reasonably anticipate that their basis of motivation will be intelligible to others. The logic of this anticipation is not a private knowledge of formal structure but rather a lived participation in expansively social networks of perception, convention, and meaning. In the presence of a standard, we *know* signs because others know them too, and we learn signs by witnessing a small fragment of their history as social objects. All signs are arbitrary because all signs exist in the present as the faded descendants of an original, authentic self that can no longer be traced directly. All signs are iconic because they are brought into real-time discourse as acts of recreation from memory. It is this double presence that builds the intimate simultaneity between speakers and hearers in a particular here-and-now.

What drives the standardization of NSL is thus not an attempt to configure the relationship of words and things along particular logics of mutual patterning but rather a very characteristic engagement with the social dimensions of linguistic provenance. What makes *long* signing different from *short* signing, simply, is the fact that *long* signing uses forms that iterate transparently against a particular moment of creation in the meetings of the NSL National Development Committee. These meetings thus serve an important originary function, parallel to but distinct from what the Vedas offer hearing language. In the context of broader South Asian engagements with linguistic form, the character of this distinction is telling. By focusing their attention not on the formal structure of signs but rather on the social networks through which signs route, deaf activists in Nepal assemble a logic of origin for everyone and everything deaf. NSL becomes, in this sense, a vanishing point for deaf Nepal's own constituted history. Though hearing language may exist today only as the echoes of some long-forgotten past, NSL is always there to be remembered at the intersection of deaf and hearing worlds.

BAKERY MANDATES

The Bakery Cafe is Kathmandu's largest restaurant chain and, according to its website, it "introduced fast food culture to the Kathmandu valley."

In addition to its assorted fried doughs and fatty snacks, the chain is well known for employing at most of its branches an entirely deaf wait staff. This is conspicuously advertised: upon entering the restaurant, patrons are greeted with a sign that reads, "Please use Sign Language with our staff. Thanks for caring" (figure 18).

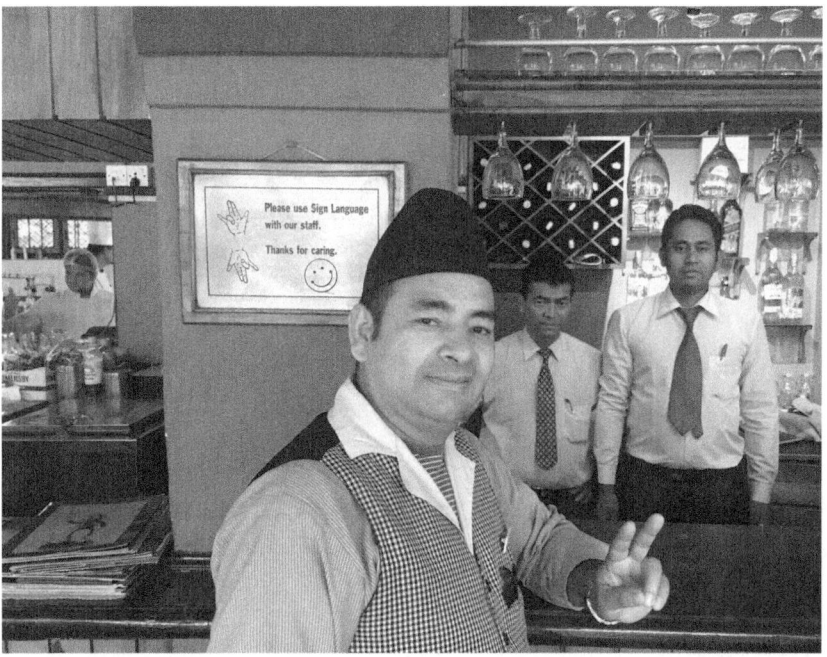

Figure 18. Staff at the Bakery Cafe in Baneshwar, Kathmandu

This request plays fast and loose with the idea of linguistic competency generally and sign language competency in particular, of course. Very few nondeaf people in Nepal know how to sign in any real sense of the word, and those who do certainly don't need to be instructed to do so. But, as the first thing that greets customers as they enter the restaurant, this message has far-reaching implications for its hearing audience: to participate in the modern multilingualism of junk food high cuisine, one must be ready to communicate with the deaf. To these ends, the idea that sign language might be something that everyone *already knows* is both palpable and powerful. Whatever the notice's broader intentions, however, there is no question that its request is meant to be taken very literally. The restaurant's expansive menu is organized into long columns of print much too small to be pointed at precisely with blunt fingers. At some branches, the menus are even laminated to the table under a thick sheet of glass. Given the meticulous attention to detail that accompanies every other aspect of the restaurant's customer experience, it is hard to imagine that this attempt to push customers into signing is even slightly accidental. At the Bakery Cafe, you will sign, or you will starve.

And it works. Only very occasionally, in my experience, will patrons call over a hearing manager, break out a pen and paper, or otherwise somehow "cheat" by summoning the aid of external supports. As they order food and negotiate payment, the patrons of the Bakery Cafe experience themselves as participating effectively in sign language. The particulars of this process have already been sketched at various points over the past two chapters, so I won't belabor the role of the hearing here. In broad terms, however, signs are made in the Bakery Cafe along the very same lines that organize effective communication between the deaf and the hearing everywhere. On several instances, for example, I saw patrons order a pizza by indicating a round object that is cut into sectors, or alternately by forming a triangular shape and then indicating that it should be eaten pointy-end first. Dosas, meanwhile, were sometimes referenced by their long cylindrical shape and other times by the rolling process that is used to produce them. What's being shared here is not an arbitrary categorical knowledge of signifiers and signifieds but instead a shared phenomenology of salience, cultivated as an intersubjective sensibility of what it is about objects that make them distinct.

What I find most interesting, however, and what is potentially crucial to the way we think about the problem of language generally, is what happens next. Once the hearing have made their snack preferences effectively known, their NSL-fluent waiter must return to the kitchen to pass the request on to the NSL-fluent cook. There, the waiter will often communicate the order not with fixed conventional signs but rather by reproducing the ad hoc gesture made moments prior by the nonsigning patron. This is unexpected, to say the least. Every item on this menu has a well-established corresponding lexical form, and every cook and every waiter who works at the Bakery Cafe knows each and every one of them. Indeed, given the specialized character of this vocabulary, it is entirely likely that these words originated here among this staff. Nevertheless, when waiters report their orders to the kitchen, they demonstrate a marked preference for recreating the formal contours of their earlier discursive encounter with the nonsigner. This preference comes at the expense of everything most fundamental to hearing language, including especially the idea of a vocabulary constituted by a specifically deaf linguistic knowledge.

This choice is especially conspicuous because these are exactly the circumstances that we would typically expect to organize the most normative and lexically oriented forms of signing: (1) highly proficient signers who know each other well, (2) communicating about a subject matter fully elaborated in the standard lexicon, (3) in a context wholly organized around the effective transmission of a specific and narrow body of information. These same waiters have been placing orders of these same fifty food items with these same cooks for sometimes a decade or more. Though the deaf must often be very creative to communicate effectively with others, this is the context for deaf Nepal where communicative efficacy is perhaps least complicated.

I do not have a simple explanation for why signers often choose to sign this way. A fixed vocabulary would no doubt provide a far easier basis of communication in a busy kitchen, so it would seem an extraordinarily strange choice to instead recreate the actions of hearing people in context. Nevertheless, when I asked waiters about why they chose to sign in this way, they tended to have very little by way of a reply. Some said they couldn't remember having done it, and others just shrugged and explained that's how signing works. Most seemed uncomfortable that I was asking these questions at all, a consequence, I suspect, of my position as a researcher interested in their language. Employment is often very difficult for the deaf to come by, and anything that allows one to work indoors in particular carries with it significant prestige. Not coincidentally, the staff of the Bakery Cafe are more likely than average to be influential players in the politics of deaf Kathmandu. With this prominence, however, comes a certain vulnerability, felt as a responsibility to represent the whole of the deaf community in public contexts. Any implication likewise that a signer is deviating from preferred forms of language is prone to be taken as a criticism, implying that he or she is capable only of "short" and nothing more. At the Bakery Cafe and elsewhere, when I asked about linguistic practices that I was surprised to see, I often found myself subject to lectures about the importance of the NSL dictionary, lectures that could only be described as rehearsed.

It was never my intention to put anyone on their guard, of course. To the contrary, the capacity that deaf people share to draw the hearing effectively into deaf ways of communicating is to my mind far more interesting and far more productive as a kind of unity than any list of standard word-forms could ever be. Indeed, the fact that deaf people can incorporate the clumsy gestures of hearing would-be signers into a fluent knowledge of signing is about the most impressive display of linguistic virtuosity I can imagine. It illustrates, to use Frank Bechter's term (Bechter 2009), a culture of "conversion," by which hearing things are made deaf through a process of appropriation and reorganization. In technical terms, these practices would appear to be driven by an intuition that the primary constituent of linguistic structure is, of all things, *reported speech*, though with the thunderously large caveat that what is getting *reported* here is not actually *speech* in any conventional sense of the word. These preferences for complexly motivated recreations of past moments of discourse show up throughout the conversations of highly fluent signers: as gossip, street directions, political strategizing, descriptions of sitcom episodes, and the most idle forms of banter. In other words, the choice I am characterizing here to use hearing gestures as *words* in fluent speech is not the consequence of an exceptional context motivating exceptional kinds of language. It is instead a choice so familiar that both waiters and cooks can make it without even realizing it at the end of a ten-hour shift.

The NSL dictionary offers to deaf worlds a founding moment of their own, parallel to but ultimately separate from the acoustic ontologies of the hearing Vedas. Nevertheless, the dictionary's capacity to organize ways of remembering a shared linguistic history is not singular. Instead, the deaf would seem to orient around numerous such lexical horizons, some materially institutionalized in books and other so fleetingly ephemeral that they disappear at the end of each customer's meal. What drives the structure of language in this context is not reducible to a correspondence between meaning and form. Rather, meaning and form are themselves the consequences of a very particular kind of intersubjective agency. In these moments, words are made present for others as the memories of past experiences shared. It is here that we find a common thread unifying signing in all of its diverse manifestations, reaching through the Bakery Cafe at one extreme and passing back to even very isolated signers at another. When Mahesh (described in chapter 3) first established reference to his cooking pot, for example, he did so on the basis of our mutual engagements with vision and touch. As soon as our pot-handle sign became fixed enough to become citable in its own right, however, it acquired a local scope of arbitrariness that pushed these phenomenological organizations into the background. Later, when the deaf leaders and I used words drawn from NSL's conventional vocabulary, we were invoking threads of citation that extended beyond the present context of discourse to a standard we all knew. Though perdurant communities of speech are a necessary condition of the kinds of fixed lexical forms represented in the NSL dictionary, fixed lexical forms are themselves not a necessary consequence of communities of speakers. Far from presuming a shared knowledge of fixed signs, signers engage interlocutors on the basis of nuanced estimations of perception and memory.

As a way of explaining these dynamics, I would propose a different approach to the problem of linguistics motivation. All signs are arbitrary to the extent that they harken back to memories of the past, and all signs are iconic to the extent that they carry forward on the basis of similarity to past forms. These are not descriptive facts about signs but rather a relationship that emerges between signers in the present. To distinguish signs as simply iconic or arbitrary in their own right, then, is to erase the most basic organizing properties of NSL's form. To find a new account of NSL's perdurance over time, we need a new account of linguistic motivation as well.

What I propose is a logic of vectors, where every word is a showcase of its past (cf. Basso 1988). Signers draw interlocutors into alignments of intelligibility, built on presumptions about the webs of referential history that may or may not be known by an other. The formal regularities exhibited by NSL speakers are thus better attributed to an elaborate and nuanced sensitivity to citational semiosis. Words, in this sense, are not the repositories of a particular specified content frozen in time, but rather act as the projection of lived histories of language use into an emergent present. What is critical is that these vectors of citation may draw from both the perceptual intuitions shared between speakers in context, on the one hand, and variously larger or smaller circumscriptions of the NSL speech community, on the other. A more arbitrary sign like MONDAY might be tied to a very particular moment of naming, relevant and accessible only to a narrow group with a shared institutional memory, whereas a more accessible sign like BUFFALO might draw from iconic inventories that are not strictly linguistic. Expressive forms can emerge and disappear in the span of a single exchange, passing forward only as the traces of a shared history of experience. Lexical signs and gestural signs, in this sense, are actually the same kind of thing, though they evoke different histories of discourse.[8] All signs, likewise, are ultimately anaphoric within a vast imagined landscape of all possible previous speech, not just as a property of semantic reference but also as a condition of their very form. What signers speak—whether with the hearing or with each other—is a language of citation.

In these terms, we can understand both language standardization projects and code-focused models of linguistic structure as attempts to empower very particular experiences of language as a presence in the world. In each case, what is at stake is the possibility that a particular technique of intelligibility should serve as the basis of linguistic objecthood most broadly. For the teachers of NSL and the writers of its dictionaries, the idea is to route all legitimate speech through citational histories tracing back to a vanishing point in the deaf institutions of Kathmandu. According to this framework, what makes NSL intelligible is not any particularity of structure but rather its embeddedness in an identified speech community with a shared collective memory. The opposition of "language" and "gesture" may serve the needs of linguistic analysis, but this distinction is ultimately no less rooted in institutional histories than the distinctions between "short" and "long" are. Perceptually sensitive linguistic practices cannot be described in perceptually naïve terms, and accounts of form will not suffice when imposed upon signers attentive to the processes by which things come to be. What characterizes modern NSL is not its iconic or arbitrary modalities as such but rather the potential for passage between them as a deliberate way of managing the scope of everything that is intelligible about words.

Of course, this problem of intelligibility goes both ways. The Bakery Cafe, as one of the earliest and best-known examples of the new public spaces that host Nepal's aspirational middle class, is an ideal place to be seen by others. Though its appeal to "fast food culture" is tied to explicitly Euro-American aesthetic sensibilities, the Bakery Cafe was also one of the first midtier restaurants to

---

8.   Notably, formal linguistics has recently demonstrated increased interest in the historical basis of linguistic form. Juliette Blevins's work in *Evolutionary Phonology* (2004), for example, explains the strong typological trends evident in the world's languages as evidence not of cognitive organizations, as the field has traditionally argued, but rather of low-level perceptual and articulatory biases that accumulate in formal structures probabilistically. Though the present book does not explicitly engage questions of phonological form in sign language, I remain deeply indebted to Blevins's work as a way of thinking about linguistic pasts and presents.

market directly to a Nepali (rather than a tourist) clientele. This is, in other words, a place that is all about performing the recreation, reorientation, and translation of categories.

In particular, the Bakery Cafe has a reputation as an ideal place to take a date. Many of the young couples I interviewed made it a point to mention that they really liked the inclusion of the deaf in particular. They liked, they said, that patronizing the restaurant could be seen as charitable. They felt that the deaf needed opportunities for self-advancement, and they liked feeling more progressive than their parents in this regard. This was only part of the appeal, however. Many also added that the fact of an entirely deaf floorstaff caused the restaurant to feel what they called, using the English word, "private." In this, they were referring, I think, to the sense of intimacy in public made possible by the restaurant's loud music and waiters who can't overhear your conversation. In this space, it is possible to sit close to a pretty girl or handsome boy and to talk about wonderful secret things without having to worry that they will be overheard by the daughter of your mother's coworker's brother. What the Bakery Cafe sells in this regard is a controlled kind of intimacy, consequentially external to the suffocating impositions of kinship that are more familiar to life in Kathmandu. One young woman, perhaps aged nineteen or twenty, said that she liked coming to the Bakery Cafe because she felt like she and her boyfriend were completely alone in the universe when they were here. Amidst the deaf waiters, the abundance of white noise, and the strategically arranged tables and booths, there was no one around to hear and repeat what they said. She seemed so delighted by this experience of boundedness, in fact, that I didn't have the heart to tell her that her waiter was a man named Dinesh whose parents had sent him to Calcutta for primary school, where he was trained in lipreading. He was, as a consequence, one of the very few people in town who could hear her from across the noisy restaurant floor.

CHAPTER 6

Laxmi: The properties of people

Wholly occupied with discernible and present objects and with the few ideas he had acquired by the eye, he did not even draw comparisons among the ideas he seemed to have taken in. It's not that he naturally lacked mind; but the mind of a man, when deprived of the intercourse of others, is so little stimulated and so little cultivated that he never thinks except when necessarily forced by external objects.

– Georges-Louis Leclerc, comte de Buffon, *Natural History: General and Particular*, vol. 3, chapter 7: "Of the Sense of Hearing"

THE DEAF MUTE SPEAKS!

From the airport, the quickest way to Thirbam Sadak on foot is through the Pashupati temple complex. One day, I was passing through that area with Laxmi KC, a prominent figure in deaf Kathmandu, who serves on both the Nepali Sign Language National Development Committee and the Deaf Women's Committee. She had met me that morning at the airport, and we were on our way to an important budget meeting when an unexpected *chakka jam* (vehicle strike) had risen up to foil our best intentions. Though much of the city shuts down during *chakka jams*, deaf organizations often don't. When I asked Laxmi why this was so, she speculated that deaf people must not hear the announcement. I suspect she was only mostly kidding.

Having cut through the temple grounds, we stopped in a densely populated central market space above the cremation *ghats*, below the *linga* shrines, and across from the pilgrim hotels and the bus park. Laxmi was texting furiously in hopes of persuading some generous soul to come pick us up. These were big favors she was calling in. Those who drive during *chakka jams* risk seeing their cars vandalized or worse, but Laxmi insisted that she had important business at this meeting. If it took place without her, she explained, her work could be set back significantly. It was several miles uphill to the NFDH offices, and we were already late. Where we stood waiting, we were surrounded by several hundred people, mostly pilgrims from across South Asia, interspersed by the flock of merchants eager to sell them things. Buyers protested bitterly at the inflated rates for fruit, colored powders, confections, and ritual tokens, but business was booming nevertheless in several different currencies. Amidst this throng of trade also stood some of the complex's many devotees, split roughly evenly between the Brahmins in their immaculate robes and the sadhu renunciates covered in cremation ash.

As I signed with Laxmi about our dilemma, an elderly man approached us, staring and uncomfortably close. He was dressed in what would have been the height of fashion thirty years prior: tight pants of natural cotton and a dark tailored jacket, both of which were clean and recently pressed. As a striking counterpoint, he was chewing on a truly massive mouthful of *pān*, the sloppy amalgam of herbs, betel leaves, and areca nuts known for yielding copious quantities of bright red saliva. Laxmi didn't seem to be bothered by his proximity or constant spitting, but I was distracted. Sign language often attracts gawkers, and relegating their attentions to the background was a skill that I had only barely begun to acquire at this point my fieldwork. Seeing the difficulty I was having, Laxmi turned her back to block his view. Undeterred, he shifted his position and watched us for a few more minutes, quizzical but smiling. Abruptly, he waved down a nearby woman who I presume was his wife. As she approached, he grabbed her by the arm and pulled her over to us. "Look! The foreign mute is talking to the Nepali mute. That is how they talk!" He grinned broadly as the woman beside him grew increasingly embarrassed. Hoping naïvely that he would go away, I smiled and said, addressing him as uncle: "I'm not actually deaf, you know." At this, his jaw dropped. He turned to his wife once again and proclaimed, "*Arre!* The foreign mute can even speak Nepali!"

Though he delivered his punchline with expert timing, I don't know that our new acquaintance ever actually caught the joke. Laxmi's colleagues at the meeting found it hilarious, however, and we were asked to retell the story at least a half dozen times once we'd finally arrived. The participants waiting at the packed budget meeting—which included virtually everyone of political import in deaf Kathmandu—were initially grumpy at our tardiness, but this story was the perfect peace offering; it was the kind of thing that everyone could laugh about, but more importantly it demonstrated and reaffirmed the basis of solidarity that drives so much of deaf activism. Every deaf person has tales of misrecognition like this one, and the act of recounting these shared experiences is an excellent way to smoothe over the interpersonal tensions inherent in political work. What this old man at the temple offered us was a parable about the hearing ignorance of deaf lives, one that inverts the normally very clear stakes of naïve irony. Because the deaf must constantly grapple with judgments laid upon them by the hearing, there is a great deal of cynical pleasure to be had in finding evidence to suggest that the hearing cannot even manage a coherent account of the principles by which they judge. This was, in short, a discursive comeuppance, one of many in a long chain that shapes the logic of deaf political life. For reasons that should be obvious but apparently aren't, of course *lāṭos* do not speak Nepali. Even a *lāṭo* could tell you that.

Nevertheless, the absurdity of speaking mutes is evidently more intelligible in context to deaf activists than it is to hearing pilgrims. This is perhaps no surprise. The deaf spend their lives honing a nuanced attention to the material properties of voice, and with this practice come strong, explicit understandings of the conditions, consequences, and implications of voice's presence. Only within a naïve perceptual framework could something like this joke float by unseen. In these moments, what the hearing demonstrate is just how sticky identity can be: signers are apparently so mute that they remain mute even when they do the one thing that mutes by definition cannot. What makes this nonperception possible are the powerfully specific phenomenological asymmetries that characterize the landscape shared by the hearing and the deaf. Words are obstinate things. They allow people to pass through otherwise obvious contradictions of meaning simply by the inertia of their presence. Consequently, though I sympathize with the general instinct to lampoon the hearing in service of deaf political identity, I also suspect that there was a great deal more going on at Pashupati than mere slow-wittedness.

To appreciate the perceptual nuances that make this act of misengagement possible, we must pay attention to the particularities of the phrasing involved:

"*Kuire lāṭo nepāli pani bolna sakdo rahechha*" (The foreign mute can even speak Nepali!). From its start, the statement invokes a double dose of epithets—*kuire* and *lāṭo*—each of which is more colloquial and provocative than the English gloss "foreign mute" does justice. As previously discussed, the word *lāto* (lit., "mute") is a problem for the deaf. They consider it pejorative, though it is not usually intended as such per se by nondeaf speakers in any given instance of utterance. By calling Laxmi and me *lāto*, however, the man at Pashupati was tying us in with a discursive history of insults, even if he didn't necessarily know how to talk about us in any other way. The other word, *kuire* (lit., "foggy", a reference to eye-color rather than skin), treads through many of the same ambivalences, though of course the power dynamics of foreigners and deaf people in Nepal are so radically different as to make comparisons of their relative stakes as nomenclature fairly useless. As epithets, however, both *kuire* and *lāṭo* function as exclamation points as much as meanings. They align attentions in the here-and-now by organizing a shared experience of something strange, sealed in this particular expression by the man's use of the verb *rahechha*. This word's infinitive form—*rahanu*—means simply "to remain" or "to continue to be," but as it is inflected here it serves more as an evidential marker, one indicating that the information being conveyed was only recently discovered by the speaker. In literal and thus clumsy terms, the implication is something like "I have recently learned that it was always the case." This is, in other words, an experience of others regimented by time. Nepali-speaking foreign mutes are a surprise, but the surprise is the fact that they have been there all along.

This man at Pashupati was not, in other words, merely describing people in the world in order to communicate information about them. He was narrating his own experience of them as it unfolded before him, and his first instinct upon realizing that he had noticed something unusual was to bring his wife nearby so that she could experience it too. In this, he was extending his subjective observations into an intersubjective alignment, one that he would perhaps even share with others in his community long after they had returned home. This is a familiar ambition of tourism, religious or otherwise. Here in Kathmandu, the world is filled with surprising things, and sharing that surprise with others is a powerful way for groups of people to know one another.

Understood in these terms, we can begin to see this man's reaction as revealing more than just incoherence. Specifically, I would like to suggest that the relevant descriptive categories at stake here emerged from patterns of seeing organized chiefly by time. Because tall Caucasians are more visibly conspicuous in crowded temple squares than signers are, the *kuire* became present before the *lāṭo* did. Two distinct revelations thus unfolded in sequence: first, the foreigner was mute, and most foreigners aren't mute; second, the foreigner spoke Nepali, and most foreigners don't speak Nepali. The fact that these two alignments converged upon a single person was noteworthy as a matter of coincidence, but as a phenomenological experience it seems not necessarily the case that each contradicted the other. A third possible revelation—that mutes can speak—slipped between the cracks of salient perception entirely. In other words, though the world elaborated here stipulates three distinct properties mapped to a body—foreignness, muteness, and Nepali-speaking—it is a mistake to presume from the outset that all properties must resolve upon the object of perception that hosts them simultaneously. It is a mistake, specifically, to presume that characteristics always come *after* the people they characterize.

Framed in these terms, we begin to see the asymmetry inherent in what this man experienced: this was a story about a foreigner who was mute and also Nepali-speaking, but—critically—it was not a story about a mute who was Nepali-speaking and foreign. According to naïve forms of analysis, this is an obvious paradox, but if we begin with the assumption that statements about the equivalence of two things *do* something rather than merely *describe* something, the processes at stake in these kinds of interactions take on a new ethnographic urgency. Specifically, they reveal an especially deaf kind of problem. Because the deaf are in a constant state of being discovered by a hearing public—because, ultimately, narratives about them are so entangled by locally organized phenomenological orientations—the question of personhood itself comes to rest on the unfolding of presence and predication in real-time practice. In a world filled unevenly with *lāṭos*, *kuires*, and *kuire lāṭos*, what does it mean for someone to be two things at once?

BEING LAXMI, HERE AND THERE

Whatever else they may say, everyone agrees that Laxmi KC is remarkable. In the many conversations that I witnessed about her, three claims consistently came up: first, in school, all of the boys were infatuated with her; second, she does not speak much but neither is she shy; and third, she has no acquaintances, but only friends and enemies. This last point in particular was often delivered with an intentionally melodramatic edge, pitching the world into jagged alliances and animosities almost worthy of a soap opera. Though deaf Nepal, like any other community, has its share of political divisions and personal rivalries, this articulation of friction as itself constituting the social order is atypical. Laxmi—to be blunt—is polarizing. According to her many friends, she is a fiercely loyal and powerfully effective ally. Everyone has a story about what she can do, whether it's persuading intransigent people, fixing broken machines, or recovering stolen property. One woman even told me that Laxmi made her husband stop drinking. According to her many detractors, however, Laxmi is always looking for a fight and takes great pleasure in humiliating those who oppose her. Everyone agrees that she is exceptionally brilliant.

Laxmi has worked for more than a decade at what is arguably the country's most prestigious travel agency. This is unusual. Many deaf people have jobs, of course, but typically they work behind closed doors in menial and anonymous trades. Laxmi's labor, however, sits on the front lines of hearing customer service. In the course of her employment, she has met countless celebrities and even a few heads of state. She is a conspicuously visible part of her company, and I'll admit that I was initially quite cynical about the motivations behind this prominence. After all, a great deal of tourism in Nepal is organized at the intersections of ecological splendor, cultural exotics, and the innocence of the poor (Adams 1996). More than one village has found itself dropped from the tour routes simply because its inhabitants are no longer authentic enough (read: economically marginal enough) to offer a powerful experience. As a hedge against these risks, the presence of a deaf woman in an upwardly mobile position of professional labor might be very strategic, offering a heartfelt story about constraint and survival that would no doubt resonate with many wealthy tourists. There is no question, I think, that Laxmi has been mobilized in exactly these terms to the service of her company's brand. Her boss is adamant, however, that this motivation for him only goes so far. Ultimately, he says, Laxmi is successful because "she knows what her clients want before they do and because she is very good at making those things happen." This is a standard line in the tourism business, but I suspect here he actually means it. He notes how effectively she can communicate though writing and carefully managed eye-contact, and he says that he understands this ability of hers as a sign of deep intelligence. Though Laxmi, like all deaf people, sometimes finds herself serving more as a category than an individual, there is no question among anyone who works with her that she is charismatic, dedicated, and fiercely effective.

I had been eager to interview Laxmi since the first time I met her, and I hoped to trace out her unusual biography to better understand questions of deaf gender identity in particular. During my first few field visits, she simply declined. Years later, however, much to my surprise, unprompted she agreed to talk. For nearly six months, we tried and failed to find a time to meet. With anyone else, I would have taken so many false starts as a sign that my request was being politely and indirectly declined. This explanation didn't really fit Laxmi, however, who I believe would without hesitation not only turn down my requests explicitly but also explain (probably in public) why I should have known better than to ask in the first place. Instead, the problem seemed to be entirely logistical. Laxmi works long and unpredictable hours, and, on the few occasions we did manage to meet at KAD, our plans to talk were foiled by the arrival of someone "too gossipy." Maintaining a proper degree of confidentiality is important to Laxmi. She talks about it often, and she agreed to speak to me, she said, because she trusted my ability to remain discreet.[1] Nevertheless, the hazards of sign language are such that you can never really know who might be watching in. It would be far better, she ultimately suggested, if I just came to her house on a Saturday convenient to us both.

Laxmi lived at the time on the outskirts of the Kathmandu Valley in a farmhouse situated at the intersection of a twelfth-century Newar hamlet, an eighteenth-century Chhetri village, and a growing number of twenty-first-century residential "colonies." When I arrived at the bus stop that Laxmi had identified for me, I proceeded to the corner store she told me to go to. From there, she instructed, I should ask where she lived and someone would direct me to her house. When I made my first inquiries, however, the shopkeeper was reluctant to tell me anything. I initially assumed she was protecting Laxmi, who is young and unmarried and thus to be shielded from anonymous male visitors. I explained that, as I understood it, Laxmi's father would also be home, but, if that turned out not to be the case, perhaps somebody could bring her here instead so that we could talk in one of the public teashops nearby. The shopkeeper apologized for any distrust she had implied and made her hesitations more explicit: Laxmi's father was himself the problem. He was

---

1. Including by obscuring her identity in anything I wrote.

a difficult neighbor, you see. Interactions with him typically didn't end well, particularly if money was involved. She didn't want to get into specifics, but before I proceeded to the house she wanted to make sure that I understood whom I was dealing with. I didn't, of course, but I thanked her for the warning and headed on.

As I approached the house, Laxmi came out onto the road to greet me. She asked after my parents and grandparents and then directed me to a small paved courtyard behind a tidy brick-and-tile building. There, a middle-aged man sat in a small patch of sun on a grass mat. His face had three or four days of stubble and he wore a traditional Nepali outfit, a *daura suruwal*, that was frayed and dingy in sharp contrast to Laxmi's modest but meticulous self-presentation. Laxmi uttered a single sign, "father," and motioned for me to sit on another grass mat nearby. At this, she disappeared into the house. Laxmi's father, meanwhile, was shuffling through a tangled stack of newsprint. I greeted him, as is convention, by asking if he had eaten yet today. He looked at me for a moment over his thick plastic-rimmed glasses, but otherwise didn't acknowledge my question. Instead, over what I experienced as an extremely uncomfortable several minutes of silence, he proceeded to reassemble his stack of pages into three distinct newspapers—one royalist, one centrist, and one Maoist. When he was finished, he creased them carefully and placed them in a row in front of me. He nodded and opened his palm slightly, a gesture that I would have understood in other circumstances as permission to proceed. I had no idea what I was supposed to do.

Though I am still frequently disoriented by social cues in Nepal, I had never experienced anything quite so disorienting as this. I am sure that I began to stammer something about my purpose there, but Laxmi's father cut me off abruptly with a question: "Dialectic *bhaneko ke ho, bhana ta babu?*" (Tell me son, what does *dialectic* mean?). Because he had used the English word "dialectic" in an otherwise Nepali question, I assumed he was looking for a translation. I responded hesitantly with a guess and hoped that I was right: "*Vivādatā*," I said. I wasn't right, really. *Vivādatā* sometimes passes as a gloss for "dialectic" in Nepali Marxist circles, though any technical sense is generally drowned out by the word's more colloquial meaning along the lines of "conflict," "opposition," or even just "disagreement." In hindsight, a better answer would have been "*Dvandavād*," but in any case it seems that proper translations were not really the issue here because Laxmi's father made no effort to correct me. Instead, he just shook his head, obviously annoyed. "*Sabda thāhā chha, tara kurā bhaneko ke ho?"* (I know the word, but what does the idea mean?). When I hesitated, he answered for me: *"Jaba eutā kurā ra tyas ko ulto bāṭa nayā kurā baninchha"* (When from one thing and its opposite a new thing is made).

The phrasing here is important, and I'll address that later, but for the moment I am more concerned with the problem of dialectics generally. This is not quite so random a topic of conversation as it might at first seem. I later learned that Laxmi's father was a Marxist politician of minor note, and he even went so far as to claim (improbably) that he had carved with his own two hands the giant hammer and sickle gracing the hillside directly above us. His interest in the dialectic was thus professional, and he was not alone in this regard. These were the early days of peace negotiations among the Maoists, monarchists, and other political parties, and the question of collaboration without self-effacement stood at the forefront of a great deal of political thought. I later noticed that the lead story in the Maoist paper in front of me was explicitly about the dialectics of power, and, though I wasn't aware of it at the time, this was presumably meant to be my prompt. For the Maoists in particular, the dialectic was at this time frequently invoked as an explicit politics of *becoming*. It framed a very real and very urgent question: What kind of a thing is a revolution after it acquires power?

At this point, Laxmi came out of the house carrying a tray with tea and biscuits. Her father was by now riffing on the failure of my American education to provide adequate attention to Marxist theory. This was, he speculated, a lingering dirty trick of Cold War politics. As he scolded me, Laxmi served what I noticed were only two cups of tea, one for me and one for her father. I realized that my ambitions to interview her had long since fallen under capture and were now being pulled in strange and unexpected directions. I implored Laxmi to sit down and talk with us. With her hands occupied by cups and kettles rendering her mute, she simply bobbed her head and pointed at her father with her chin. Once the tea had been served and her hands were her own once again, she apologized and explained that she had work to do inside. She smiled—knowingly, I think—and left me to her father's admonitions. As I had seen so many times before, deaf people in Nepal are often interested less in what things *are* and more in where they *come from*. Getting to know Laxmi was going to mean getting to know her father, and I suspect this had been the plan all along. Laxmi walked away, and I turned to face my new interview subject. He paused briefly to drink his tea as he stared into the distance down the road. I took this as an opportunity to redirect the conversation.

AUTHOR   FATHER

About sign language-

                    -about what?

Could you say something about sign language?

                    Like this? (moving hands frenetically)

Yeah

                    And what is there to say?

          (pause)

                    It's nothing. Empty talk. It's not understood.

You don't understand sign language?

                    This one's [Laxmi's]?

Indeed

                    What is there to understand? Eat this, go there, sit

                    here. This is how my daughter is. It's monkey talk.

No, no, no . . . they teach college in sign language.

You can say anything in it.

                    This is monkey talk, I said.

Nope.

          (long pause)

                    But that one [Laxmi] does good work.

What kind of work?

                    The people's struggle. She raises the awareness of

                    other deaf people.

Laxmi does?

                    Yes.

In sign language?

                    Indeed. That one is talented. We hearing-speaking

                    people can't explain "class struggle" to them, since

                    they're deaf and dumb, but that one can explain it

                    well, because the talk/thing fits ["*kurā milera*"].

It's the struggle of deaf people too, eh?

                    Yes indeed. The deaf have a "revolutionary spirit" [in

                    English]. The capitalists oppress them, but in the new

                    Nepal it will not/must not be like this.

And Laxmi helps with this?

                    She's a leader, that one.

          (Another pause, and I write some notes. Laxmi returns and I

ask her again to sit down. She declines, leaves a plate of
oranges, and returns to the house.)

> What kind of talk (*kurā*) does this one do? [Rhetori-
> cal, waves hands mockingly] Monkey talk!

Though I had heard sign language both eulogized and denigrated in these
terms countless times before, this was the first time I'd seen recognitions quite
this extreme articulated in such close proximity to each other. Laxmi's father
seemed to be portraying his daughter *simultaneously* both as a merely animal
intelligence and as a leader in the class struggle, a thing and an opposite if ever
there were one. These rapid-fire shifts in evaluative frame were difficult to make
sense of, and I found the conversation initially very disorienting. It carved a
shape of personhood for Laxmi that seemed utterly unresolvable, but as matters
unfolded I came to realize that its core disjunctions were in fact tightly organized by the different pronouns Laxmi's father used to reference his daughter.

Specifically, everything negative about Laxmi was attached to the pronoun
yo while everything positive was attached to *tyo*. *Yo* and *tyo* are both third-person
pronouns, roughly equivalent to "this" and "that" in English, though perhaps
a bit less rude when applied to people. Like "this" and "that," the distinction
between *yo* and *tyo* is generally proximity: *yo* refers to objects that are relatively
closer to a conceptual center fixed on the speaker, and *tyo* to objects relatively
farther away. This is not so much an issue of objective distance as of discursively
established contrasts in a landscape of apparent things. Here, **this** Laxmi was
tangled in monkey talk, but **that** one was leading her people to liberation. Conspicuously absent from Laxmi's father's way of referring to his daughter was
Nepali's nonspatialized third-person pronoun *u*. Though *u* is actually quite a bit
more common in general speech as a way of referencing people than either *yo*
or *tyo* are, it made no appearance in the transcript above and only an occasional
one in everything that came after. Instead, Laxmi's father spoke at length about
his daughter-near and his daughter-far.

What followed was a full three hours of this: thick Marxist exegesis paired
with wildly bifurcated assessments of Laxmi's simultaneous brute incompetence
and class heroism. What caught my attention as Laxmi's father spoke—even
before I noticed the organization of spatial pronouns that I am describing
here—was the fact that he never made any statements about what Laxmi *is* but
instead catalogued a litany of things that she was the *same as*. **This** was the same
as the prostitute widows who work near the bus park, shamed for their work but

honorable for doing what they must to survive with their children. **That** was the same as the jungle revolutionary, oppressed and unwilling to accept the ways of the capitalists. **This** was the same as a wound or injury that will never heal, since they would never afford the dowry necessary for her to marry properly. **That** was the same as a river that could not be blocked by rocks but instead inevitably wore the rocks away. **This** was the same as a monkey imitating humans. **That** was the same as Abraham Lincoln when he rallied the slaves to rebel against the capitalists. The list of equivalences went on considerably, though many of the references were completely lost on me. I don't know what it means, for example, that **this** was the same as tea but **that** was the same as coffee, nor especially that **this** is the same as a counterfeit taxi meter but **that** is the same as a taxi without a driver. Nevertheless, Laxmi's father made his claims emphatically. What emerged over time were two entirely distinct Laxmis, each attached to a different presence in space: **this** one converging on the biographically particular daughter who lived in his house and **that** one instantiating the class position borne by the universal historical dialectic.

Though some of these equivalences became convoluted enough to mire even their author at times, the logic of patterning was consistent: **this** was intimate and negative while **that** was structural and positive. These are deictic pronouns, however, which means that they work by *pointing* at something. Their meaning is not absolute but rather fixed in context upon an object of reference meant to be apparent to everyone already. If I announce at some moment that "*This* is my friend John," my statement will only make sense if everyone can see who *this* is. In similar terms, *yo* and *tyo* both presume the existence of an already apparent thing being talked about, and so we might ask about the exact identity of that thing or those things I was meant to see. In our several hours of talk, what emerged were two distinctly coherent presences, distributed over relatively closer and farther domains of space. Laxmi's father makes a great deal more sense as soon as we actually take what he says literally, recognizing that he was indeed talking about two different things—one near, one far, and both of which were his daughter in some sense of translation.

This reconfiguration of Laxmi into a daughter-near and a daughter-far carries with it some obvious problems, however. Though the notion of two irreconcilable daughters caught in a dialectic might provide some extent of satisfaction to a dyed-in-the-wool Marxist like Laxmi's father, it's not really a way to live. It is far too useful instead to occupy a world of steady things, where one always has the same number of daughters from moment to moment and where her extent of personhood is fixed to her single body. There is, in other words, an apparent disjunction between how Laxmi's father describes his daughter and how he engages with her day to day. The power of the commodity fetish—another famous dialectic—manifests precisely to the extent that it is *socially* distributed and invisible to individual participants; trying to apply it as a totality to single acts of recognition renders the entire process vacuous. Laxmi's father, however, was articulating both the most positive and most negative discourses on deafness available to him simultaneously, mapped consistently (if not always carefully) over time and space. Within this tangle, what should we understand him to mean? How can all of these things be true of a single person at once?

However wide a cultural berth we might grant to the phenomenological processes that constitute Laxmi's presence for those who know her, we are ultimately responsible to the basic fact of efficacy that Laxmi's father accomplishes in the world. He *does* know his daughter from one moment to the next. He *does* recognize her as his one and only daughter. He *does* experience a basic fact of continuity in her presence. If we are to take Laxmi's father seriously in his claim of two things that are his daughter, then we must ask: What are these things, and why are there two of them rather than one or a thousand? How does Laxmi host such polarized and seemingly irreconcilable traits? If she is both a thing and its opposite, will a novel third thing emerge from the tension within her? It's not clear. Laxmi's father lives in a world filled with many evident contradictions, but he is nevertheless a virtuoso in crafting the terms of his own perceptual frame. The moral dimensions of this framing are especially powerful in their very deliberate irresolution. It is here, perhaps, among these scattered fantasies, that we might find the truest allegory yet of being deaf in hearing worlds.

TALK/INTELLIGIBLE

Laxmi's father starts to make quite a bit more sense, I think, if we evaluate his account of two Laxmis in the terms made possible by the old man at Pashupati described earlier in this chapter. There, the figure of a speaking mute was instantiated by the unexpected convergence of "speaking" and "muteness," unified by their collocation in a single body but distinct nevertheless as presences in the world. Similarly, when Laxmi's father made his daughter intelligible in the shared discursive space between us, what he had constituted for my notice was not a person with characteristics but rather a series of manifested properties that all happen to converge at a particular time and place. When he said, at different moments, "sign language is incoherent" and "sign language is profound," for example, he was talking about exactly two different things: incoherence and profundity, both of which were more present to him as properties of the world than any ostensible convergence called "sign language" ever was. Likewise, when he talked about Laxmi and her signing, he was identifying the wide range of things he experienced in her place: incoherence, development, shame, upliftment, transformation, stasis, humanity, frivolity, and so on. What he was *not* identifying, however, was a thing called language or even a particular person named Laxmi who speaks it. As a rule, these things come later, or often even not at all.

This possibility is not so strange, perhaps. In his brilliant book *The Character of Logic in India* (1998), Bimal Krishna Matilal suggests that a similar perceptual instinct is fundamental to Sanskrit logical theory. In the Western academy, the dominant formalist tradition passing through and beyond Frege has tended to think about predicative relationships as being first and foremost "about" entities. In a statement like "Laxmi is a good leader," for example, "Laxmi" would generally stand as the more perdurant thing, extant, independently, of her ability to lead. In Indian logical traditions, however, Matilal argues that the ontology is conspicuously reversed: in this frame, the more real thing would actually be the "ability to lead," and the person we call "Laxmi" would be a functional operation of sorts, offering a spatiotemporal locus upon which a greater or lesser extent of "good leadership" (and any number of other things) might converge. Though these distinct formalizations are ultimately equivalent in narrowly semantic terms, they reveal and reiterate radically different expectations of *presence*.

In other words, it's not that Laxmi's father cannot perceive the continuity of his daughter. He can, in any number of different ways: as a biological body, as an amalgam of economic entanglements, as a chain of interrelated memories, and perhaps most of all as a presence who falls asleep each night and wakes up in the same place each morning. Nevertheless, in the course of my conversation with him, the question of these various continuities simply was not reached. It is not what felt salient or important to him in this particular configuration of time and place, and it's not what he presented to me as the thing worth noticing and talking about. Instead, by offering to our mutual engagement a series of distinct points of confluence, he was describing for me not "Laxmi" per se but rather something else entirely. Whatever this "something else" might be, it is irreducible to personhood as a preexisting mode of being. Instead, what organized Laxmi for her father—and what felt important to him to talk about—expands to incorporate a dynamic convergence of contextual configurations, each of which serves individually to position Laxmi within a distinct framing of the social world. We might say that Laxmi is a worker, a daughter, an activist, and a signer, for example, but we might just as reasonably say that work, daughterhood, activism, and signing all converge upon the place that makes her be. Monkey talking and class heroism both converge on her too, apparently, but these are different attributions that occur in quite literally distinct articulations of place.

In a recent article, Judith Farquhar (2012) describes a similar descriptive intervention by a medical scholar named Dr. Lu. For Dr. Lu, acts of reference offer a way to interrelate multiple, coexisting, often incompatible ontologies, essential to the effective practice of medicine. When faced with an impossible simultaneity of Western and Chinese pathological modalities, for example, simply talking with a patient about a symptom in context serves to displace the problem of disjunction into a more productive intersubjective alignment. This way of engaging with others through the discursive constitution of things mutually apparent is for Dr. Lu not only a kind of experiential phenomenon but, moreover, a basic condition of the social world. The countervailing notion, that people and things should stand still to be referenced, is perhaps the more peculiar intellectual commitment after all.

As it turns out, Laxmi's father was telling me this all along. Though he does not share Dr. Lu's technical vocabulary—nor especially the Chinese notion of *duixiang* ("object," or, as a more literal alternate suggested by Farquhar, "the image we face")—his descriptive account of the Laxmi-he-knows similarly anticipates both emergence and perdurant form to coexist in time. To understand his sense of Laxmi in these terms, however, we must begin by understanding what he means when he entails her as a presence before him. Given his posture as a self-conscious intellectual, his definition of the dialectic would seem to offer a particularly good roadmap to this task: "*Jaba eutā kurā ra tyas ko ulto baṭā nayā kurā baninchha*" (When from one thing and its opposite a new thing is made). The phrasing here should be familiar at first glance, but nevertheless the particularities of its expression are steeped in local categories that my translation fails utterly to convey. By tracing these nuanced contours out, the stakes of Laxmi's deafness reveal an entirely new shape.

For starters, the idea that the synthesized "new thing" is *made* implies precisely the wrong history. The Nepali verb—*baninchha*—is morphologically configured to suggest a transformation with ambiguous agency and timing. It is perhaps better glossed as "occurs" or "comes to be" in many circumstances, though even these translations carry with them telic and temporal implications that are wholly inappropriate to context. Indeed, as discussed in the previous chapter's account of the ahistoricity of sound, the possibility of realization without agentive cause is central in much of South Asian philosophy to the phenomenon of being itself. In these same terms—against European theorists who have tended to identify the *synthesis* of a dialectic as an output or emergence within a fundamentally historical process—Laxmi's father is identifying something with no clear beginning or end. He projects upon his daughter his experience of both leadership and incompetence, but he doesn't need these incompatible properties to resolve across time for the "new thing" to be made. Instead, by constituting his dialectic as a spatiotemporal convergence, he is describing his daughter's emergence in context from the perspectival alignment of things that have been there all along. He is describing, in other words, a tension in his own acts of seeing. Laxmi *always* exists as the potential of both her myriad forms and her unification, but the person who becomes consequential is ultimately the one (or several) that he and I experience together.

It is in these same terms that we should understand *kurā*, the Nepali word I have translated above as "thing." This is a flimsy equivalence at best. In English, the word "thing" is the quintessential generic container, but it is nevertheless far too mired in cultural particularity to serve adequately in a Nepali context of reference. A *kurā* is indeed a thing, but it is not a thing like English things nor even Dr. Lu's *duixiang*. We could certainly specify that there are many different *kurā* for sale in a particular store, for example, but we could just as easily say that a pandit's *kurā* is hard to understand because it depends too much on technical jargon. To do *kurā* (*kurā garnu*) is "to talk" in the most general sense, but yet a person's *kurā* refers not to his or her aggregated acts of speech but rather to the intentions and ideas they contain. *Kurā* is furthermore a general term for language itself, such that we might distinguish between Gurung *kurā*, English *kurā*, and Nepali *kurā*. When pressed into translation, *kurā* is sometimes glossed as "thing," sometimes as "talk," and sometimes as "idea," but of course this trifurcated analysis into English does not imply the existence of three distinct modes of being in a Nepali context.[2] Instead, *kurā* forces us into a single, unexpected object frame: talk/idea/thing.

---

2.   See the "kurāgraphy" of Desjarlais (2003, 19), for a more comprehensive inventory of *kurā*'s forms.

This convergence of language, thought, and being has complex implications, especially in light of Matilal's metaphysics described above. Just as talk is real by virtue of its ability to manifest the echoes of being as a *presence* in the here-and-now (cf. chapter 5), we might regard "things" as existing to the extent that they host a diversity of abstract categories in a domain of experience. In these terms, *kurā* is perhaps best understood most broadly as an *attribution* to time and space; whether it is an attribution of material characteristics, semantic meanings, or the traces of a social history is ultimately secondary to its broader consequentiality as a basis of lived experience. What *kurā* describes, in other words, is an object—and, simultaneously, a process of objecthood—that exists through its capacity to create shared moments of encounter between social actors.

My goal here is not to assert any crude isomorphism between Nepali words and Nepali thought but rather to suggest that the English descriptive terminology carries with it far more theoretical baggage than we might realize. Indeed, throughout this book, the deaf have demonstrated just how contextual intuitions can be about what it means to say that "things" like people exist. Laxmi's father, for his part, extends this general dilemma into an unusually explicit ethnographic frame. Specifically, his dialectic imagines a very particular interaction of things and their opposites: when the new and novel third *kurā* is produced, it is a consequence not of any historical resolution but of the shared spatial alignment of two different things simultaneously seen. In these terms, he is engaging the problem of his daughter's personhood not as an ontological fact to be recognized but rather as the ambiguous entailment of his own perception in context, encasing historical organizations of interaction within encounters with objects of the here-and-now. This is, I have argued, a condition familiar to deaf lives in Nepal. What Laxmi's father reveals for us in his definition of the dialectic, thus, is nothing less than a way of tracing the conditions of possibility for knowing the deaf. To understand him and his daughter, we must understand how he experiences the presence of *kurā*. We must understand the space of things between people that makes social worlds intelligible.

For Alfred Gell (1998), art provides people with the opportunity to do what they want to do everywhere else. This isn't so much a function of desire as it is of lived intuitions, elaborated in artistic contexts in (relatively) unfettered terms. Along these same lines, I understand Laxmi's father as an artist of sorts, basking unapologetically in his social theoretical virtuosity. Though it is well beyond my training to speculate about why he takes such pleasure in having a monkey-talking revolutionary hero for a daughter, it is evident that he does. Perhaps, in the end, no explanation is even necessary. As a daughter, Laxmi is known by her place within logics of kinship, within logics of material fact, within logics of gender, and class, and labor, and love, and rebirth. In other words, though Laxmi is knowable by the multitude of schemes she is entangled in, these schemes are not all socially equivalent. Some perdure, and some shift. Deafness is especially unstable as an attribution, and as a result all talk about Laxmi as a deaf person empowers tremendously nuanced acts of relational being. She can be a monkey talker and a revolutionary hero simultaneously to her father because, in the end, she is also his deaf daughter.

Over the course of our conversation, Laxmi's father was interested in some very technical distinctions: Did Nepal have an industrial proletariat of any significance, or was it still at a feudal stage of development? Did indigenous systems of land tenure like the *guṭhis* of the Newars or the Limbu *kipat* have revolutionary potential, or were they too backwards to be reclaimed? Among a dozen or so South Asian Marxists (about whom I knew nearly or exactly nothing), whose model of agricultural production could be best adapted to the economics of tourism? Laxmi's father approached me with a posture of unrelenting one-upmanship, but in the course of our conversation I learned some things about him as well. He had worked for several years at a light manufacturing plant, where he first encountered politics during a union-led strike. He was injured on the job somehow shortly thereafter, and he has not been able to work since. Though the precise nature of his disability was not apparent to me, he declined to elaborate when I asked. In the years that followed, he joined the central planning committees of several different communist party factions. His name had even appeared on several different ballots, but he invariably left the party before the election could happen. These relationships seem to have all faltered on interpersonal disputes (specifically, *kurā milena* = the talk/idea/thing didn't agree). Now, unable to work in any physical domain and having burned all of his bridges in politics, he has very little to occupy him beyond the memories of his ambitions and failures. This is, I think, a critical dimension of his way of engaging his daughter through me. To a nominal patriarch supported entirely by his disabled and unmarried daughter, it is no surprise perhaps that the world is filled with contradictions.

By asking me to define the dialectic for him, Laxmi's father was thus pitching our conversation into a simultaneously personal and political frame. Whatever his reasons for engaging me in this way may have been, this was a serendipitous way for him to open our conversation. The definition of the dialectic he offered was technically robust, of course, but more importantly it was also entangled by his own personal engagement with the question of his daughter. If Laxmi is indeed a third thing—and I hope it is clear that even for her father she is substantially more complex than a talking monkey or a revolutionary hero—she is a third thing very particular to his experience of her deafness. This is not, in other words, a historical materialist story about contradictions resolving in the course of time. This is not an account of conflict at all, actually. Indeed, what is perhaps most striking about the conversation I had with Laxmi's father is just how easily he seems to experience this revolutionary hero and monkey talker who is also his daughter. If we really are talking about a dialectic here, it is one manifest in the intersubjective possibilities of presence unfolding in his conversation with me. Laxmi is not a historical synthesis of contradictory terms, but rather she is the talk/thing/idea that is made/becomes/exists in the location of her body. If Laxmi is to be one person, we must explain how she is also many more. To come in to this interview as I did, expecting an already-Laxmi about whom claims could be made and to whom properties could be ascribed, is to have already missed the vast bulk of cultural work that went into making her intelligible.

In this book, I have argued that in deaf worlds the *presence* of things is most frequently and most consequentially driven not by material facts but rather by the interaction of highly patterned structures of attention in context. To see the deaf, we must see how they come to be for others in social place, or don't, and we must understand how they manage this process through a nuanced appreciation of hearing perceptions. Though questions about *being* are generally deferred to speculative philosophy, I approach them here as a distinctly *cultural* set of problems.

This space of ethnographic inquiry is not limited to deaf Nepal. It is notable, for example, that both Arjun and Laxmi are branded as *senseless* in such broadly linguistic terms. Language, with its perdurant structure and fleeting instantiation, is particularly fraught in both Euro-American and South Asian theories of being. But it is precisely this irresolvability that makes language so available to the intelligibility practices over which the deaf demonstrate mastery. When we look at Arjun's dictionary, Raghav's political speeches, Shanta Raj's *Lorem Ipsum* newspaper, Mahesh's name, and Laxmi's signs, what we see are deaf people engaged by the production of intelligible talk. But if we begin by understanding how much work is necessary to invest these objects with sense, we might ask whether they are encountered first as *talk* or first as something *intelligible*. As I have argued throughout this book, this is a question that cannot be answered without careful attention to a domain of cultural practices that usually goes unnoticed. To see the deaf, and to see perhaps many other forms of difference rooted in patterned asymmetries of perception, we must begin with an ethnographic theory grounded in the alternating presence of talk/intelligible.

Deaf lives are lived in these interstitial and unresolved spaces, and in this book I have tried to capture what this experience of contradiction is like. Through his preoccupation with the dialectic, Laxmi's father presents us with an opportunity to think about what a resolution might actually mean. This is no simple question, however. With so much of deaf cultural difference staked upon the vast gaps in hearing ways of seeing, resolution—at least for now—means effacement. It means relegating everything particular about deaf communities to a state of disengagement, negating their remarkable politics that coexists within but never settles upon hearing normative categories. Only by foregrounding these dynamics of intelligibility, then, can we begin to gauge the substance of deaf and hearing difference. This is an ambition basic to all anthropological research, and I hope that the ethnographic techniques I have described will be useful in other contexts too. For people like Laxmi, however, we should furthermore wonder whether merely *seeing* difference is ever enough. Are the radical attentions to hearing regimes of perception that I have characterized in this book satisfying as an end, or is there perhaps another future unfolding for the deaf? I'm not sure. In the weeks and months that followed my visit, I asked Laxmi many times why she wanted me to meet her father. I asked her, in other words, to give me a resolution that he failed to provide. She declined. It was only years later, under very different circumstances and in a very changed Nepal, that she showed me, in ways I could see, the first hints of her answer.

AFTER WORDS

On April 25, 2015, at 11:56 a.m., a massive earthquake struck Nepal. In all, 8,964 people died. Another three and a half million were left homeless, either by the initial destruction or by the relentless aftershocks, monsoon rains, and landslides that came in the long, traumatic months that followed.

Once primary rescue efforts had ended, the most conspicuous fact of life after the earthquake was the constant waiting. This was a relatively quiet period in the agricultural cycle for most, and, as violent aftershocks continued to threaten the country, very few were engaged in the infrastructure work that usually occupies this time. Furthermore, the government had warned citizens that anyone who began reconstruction before receiving official aid would forfeit their share, even though they would have to wait eighteen months for the first disbursement. In the interim, families improvised shelter with tarps and corrugated steel. In the temporary landscapes of this new reality, those who had not lost anyone especially close to them wrestled with very human ambivalences of scale. So many had lost so much, but this recognition was matched with a widespread perception that things could have been so very much worse. The earthquake had come on a beautiful Saturday just before noon in a part of the country that tends to work, socialize, and play outdoors. If it had happened at night or on a school day, the loss of life would have likely been an order of magnitude greater.

In Kathmandu, a majority of buildings remained standing, but the earthquake changed the landscape in other ways. Though houses generally fared well enough, nearly every unreinforced compound wall lining the city's streets was brought down, opening a world of previously interior spaces to public display. The city's lines of sight had been completely remade, and this visibility changed what it meant to live in a city with others. For months, people slept, ate, socialized, and worked in these newly revealed courtyards, as they waited for the aftershocks to quiet down and for the buildings to feel safe again.

Laxmi's house was completely destroyed, as most of the houses in her neighborhood had been. Owing to facts of wealth disparity that leave some houses more resilient than others and facts of geology that remain hidden under soil until it ceases to stand still, this part of the Kathmandu Valley experienced far more damage than the city center itself did. I saw the state of Laxmi's house when I passed through the area just a week after it had been destroyed, but it wouldn't be until almost a year later that I finally found out what happened to her. Her neighbors only knew that she didn't live there anymore. She had left two years earlier after getting married, though her father and a brother had been at home in the courtyard when the house collapsed. They had left by early the next day, however, and nobody could say for sure where they had gone.

I tried to contact Laxmi several times but never heard anything back. The consensus in the deaf community was that she was safe, but nobody I talked to had heard from her directly. Then, abruptly one morning, she messaged me over Facebook and asked if I could stop by that afternoon. She sent me a pair of GPS coordinates in an upwardly mobile neighborhood and suggested I bring some litchis when I came. When I arrived at the intersection she'd indicated, I was greeted from a balcony by her husband, a deaf man I recognized from various activism-related events around town but had never properly met. He invited me upstairs to a small, upscale apartment, where Laxmi was sitting at the dining room table sifting through a pile of trekking maps and receipts. For the next hour, the three of us caught up and traded stories. She was still with the tour company, though she was hoping to leave at the end of this coming season if she could save enough money because she wanted to have children. He had been running a small photo lab for the last fifteen years, though his fortunes had really changed only five or so years back after he retooled completely into digital, making his one of the few shops ready for the rise of smartphones in urban Nepal. They asked where I had been during the earthquake, and I said that I had taken my kids to a park in the old part of the city.

Laxmi stared for a moment at my response, then smiled. "I guess we still need to find a new sign for 'Kathmandu'," she said. It took me a moment to understand what she was talking about. The NSL sign for KATHMANDU is made with the right index finger pointing up while resting on the left palm, like a spire rising out of the earth. This is, by popular convention, a reference to Dharaharā, the early eighteenth-century watchtower that projected above the old city until the earthquake knocked it down. "They're building it again," I said. She looked skeptical. "Anyway, they built it again after it got knocked down by 1934 [the year of another devastating earthquake]." Laxmi responded dismissively: "Yes, but the city doesn't look like that anymore. Dharaharā used to tower over everything for miles, but now so many other buildings are taller."

Before I could press Laxmi on this question of linguistic aesthetics, however, I was startled by the appearance of her father as he passed into the kitchen from an occluded balcony. He had aged considerably. He had trouble walking, and the thickness of his glasses betrayed failing eyes. Laxmi responded before I could ask: "He lives here now. After the earthquake." This was an unconventional arrangement, to say the least. Most men his age would consider any extent of material dependence on the family of a son-in-law humiliating, and cohabitation with a married daughter is practically unheard of.

From the kitchen, Laxmi's father started to complain loudly about cold tea and an absence of biscuits. Laxmi must have noticed my attentions shift to the sound because she pointed her chin towards the kitchen to ask what was happening. I explained, and she bristled with irritation, "He's so selfish. It's how he's always been. All he sees is what he wants but doesn't have. The thoughts play over and over and over in his mind." My translation here fails on a few key points. To characterize how her father sees, Laxmi placed her hands at the side of her eyes like horse-blinders and then traced them forward along an increasingly narrow path. She stared down this path with eyes flitting from place to place as if searching, and she rubbed her throat with her index and middle fingers in a quickly reduplicating form of the verb LIKE while licking her lips to characterize the greediness of the appetite. She vented for a while longer. Let him buy his own biscuits, then.

All I could manage to say was, "He seems old." Laxmi's tone changed abruptly as she objected, "He's not old. He's worn thin and disappearing. He spent his whole life fighting against the oppression of laborers and peasants. He put everything into it, but they won and he lost. He lost everything." After a long pause, I told Laxmi that I'd written about her in my dissertation and that I was trying to turn it into a book. I told her that I had a chapter about the time I visited her house, when her father had had such a broad range of things to say about her and her sign language. She laughed when I told her that I'd called her Laxmi, but then got straight to the point: "Is it any good? Do your people like it?"

"Some of them do. Some also say that I need to focus my argument better."

"Too much H-A-N-D-W-A-V-I-N-G?" Laxmi smiled as she spelled out this last word in English. She had come across it, she said, in a recent editorial on an English language blog in reference to political talk. She thought it was a great commentary on hearing ways of speaking and writing generally and that it explained why, perhaps, most hearing people don't really get sign language. She added that, if I wanted to make sure that I wasn't just waving my hands, I should probably explain what my argument was so that she and her husband could judge.

I did my best, though I felt the limits of my signing at every moment. I said that the book was about how to do research on communities of people. I said that we need to understand culture if we want to understand communities, and that certain kinds of cultural difference are hard to see if we don't look for them in particular ways. Specifically, the things that people notice in the world when they interact with others is part of culture, too, and deaf people and hearing people tend to see very different things around them, especially when they're interacting with each other. Deaf people have a lot of experience evaluating what those around them do or don't perceive, I went on, and this skill is a big part of how sign language works. We talked about how her father seemed to attach to very contradictory experiences of her, for example, and I said that I thought this is why she had wanted me to meet him all those years ago. I thought that his way of seeing her—as a person, in a place, with properties and history—was extreme perhaps but also very characteristic of hearing "habits." (The sign HABIT is made by passing the blade of the right hand through a v-shape made by the left, like a skid passing through a grove.) Laxmi said she agreed. Her husband said he did too, though he was conspicuously careful not to say anything that could be construed as negative about his wife's father. We talked a bit more, and ultimately they gave me my imprimatur: if I could say all this clearly, they thought that deaf people would accept it ("accept" = two hands taking an object from in front of the body and then pulling it into the chest).

The conversation drifted to other matters, and slowly the sky started to grow dark. Abruptly, just as I was about to excuse myself to leave, Laxmi returned to her father:

> He's not a bad man. But, he talks. And when he talks, that's the thing in front of him. And he forgets about other things that are also important to him. They are over to the side. He can't see them, but they're still there. They're all pointed right at him from the side, but he sees only the talk that he is making right in front. It spins and it spins, and it's mesmerizing, and he can't look any place else to see what's there. It's there already, but he only sees the thing he's looking at.

I have balked many times throughout this book at the violence of my translations, but this statement is more inseparable from the articulatory mechanisms of signing than anything else I have tried to describe. The whole passage was perhaps ten seconds long, and its relative length as English prose is a consequence of the distinct inability that spoken languages have to articulate multiple words at once. What Laxmi established in her signing space were two distinct presences, one before her and one to the side. The one in front she identified lexically as TALK, but the one to her side remained featureless except that it was pointed right at her. She then shifted her shoulders back and forth, first to face forward and then to face from the side at the point she had occupied just a moment before. She was shifting between two roles, first one belonging to her father and then one belonging to the unnamed thing that looked at him. With these shifts in role came shifts in physicality, location, and perceptual frame. She could only see the thing she was already looking at. She went on:

People can only act on the things that are in front of them, not on the side. They don't know about those. This thing is in front here. Now what? What is it?

We deaf people face many problems. Hearing people look at us and they don't understand. This holds us down. It holds our work down. But the people who don't understand us are our families, the people in our homes. We are there in front of them. They don't understand us, but they feed us, and they help us, and they love us. And we're looking at them, and we feed them, and we help them, and we love them. . . . My father is the same. He doesn't understand but he acts. Those things you said before are true, but this is true too. This is something that you should also say. That is my request to you.

References

Ablon, Joan. 1990. "Ambiguity and Difference: Families with Dwarf Children." *Social Science & Medicine* 30 (8): 879–87.

Adams, Vincanne. 1996. *Tigers of the Snow and Other Virtual Sherpas: An Ethnography of Himalayan Encounters.* Princeton, NJ: Princeton University Press.

Alpher, Barry. 2001. "Ideophones in Interaction with Intonation and the Expression of New Information in Some Indigenous Languages of Australia." In *Ideophones*, edited by F. K. Erhard Voeltz and Christa Kilian-Hatz, 9–24. Amsterdam: John Benjamins Publishing Company.

Althusser, Louis. 1969. "Contradiction and Overdetermination." In *For Marx*, 87–128. Translated by Ben Brewster. London: Allen Lane.

Aronoff, Mark, Irit Meir, and Wendy Sandler. 2005. "The Paradox of Sign Language Morphology." *Language* 81 (2): 301–44.

Babb, Lawrence A. 1981. "Glancing: Visual Interaction in Hinduism." *Journal of Anthropological Research* 37 (4): 387–401.

Bagatell, Nancy. 2007. "Orchestrating Voices: Autism, Identity and the Power of Discourse." *Disability & Society* 22 (4): 413–26.

Bahan, Benjamin J. 2009. "Sensory Orientation." *Deaf Studies Digital Journal* 1 (1). http://dsdj.gallaudet.edu/assets/section/section2/entry19/DSDJ_entry19.pdf.

Bahira Awaj. 1998. Vol. 1.1. Kathmandu: Quality Printers.

Bakhtin, Mikhail. (1965) 1984. *Rabelais and His World.* Translated by Hélène Iswolsky. Bloomington: Indiana University Press.

Bandhu, C. M. 1989. "The Role of the Nepali Language in Establishing the National Unity and Identity of Nepal." *Kailash* 15 (3–4): 121–33.

Basso, Keith H. 1988. "'Speaking with Names': Language and Landscape among the Western Apache." *Cultural Anthropology* 3 (2): 99–130.

Bateson, Gregory. 1972. *Steps towards an Ecology of Mind*. Chicago: University of Chicago Press.

Bauman, H-Dirksen L. 2003. "Redesigning Literature: The Cinematic Poetics of American Sign Language Poetry." *Sign Language Studies* 4 (1): 34–47.

———, ed. 2008. *Open Your Eyes: Deaf Studies Talking*. Minneapolis: University of Minnesota Press.

Bechter, Frank D. 2008. "The Deaf Convert Culture and Its Lessons for Deaf Theory." In *Open Your Eyes: Deaf Studies Talking*, edited by H-Dirksen L. Bauman, 60–79. Minneapolis: University of Minnesota Press.

———. 2009. "Of Deaf Lives: Convert Culture and the Dialogic of ASL Storytelling." Ph.D. thesis, University of Chicago.

Beck, Guy L. 1993. *Sonic Theology: Hinduism and Sacred Sound*. Delhi: Motilal Banarsidass Publishers.

Bey, Hakim. (1991) 2003. *TAZ: The Temporary Autonomous Zone, Ontological Anarchy, Poetic Terrorism*. New York: Autonomedia.

Bhartṛhari. n.d. *Vākyapadīya*.

Bista, Dor Bahadur. 1991. *Fatalism and Development: Nepal's Struggle for Modernization*. Telangana, India: Orient Blackswan.

Blevins, Juliette. 2004. *Evolutionary Phonology*. Cambridge: Cambridge University Press.

Boas, Franz. 1889. "On Alternating Sounds." *American Anthropologist* 2 (1): 47–54.

———. 1940. "Decorative Designs of Alaskan Needle Cases: A Study on the History of Conventional Designs, Based on Materials in the US National Museum." In *Race, Language, and Culture*, 564–92. Chicago: University of Chicago Press.

Brentari, Diane. 1998. *A Prosodic Model of Sign Language Phonology*. Cambridge, MA: MIT Press.

———. 2008. "Establishing a Sonority Hierarchy in American Sign Language: The Use of Simultaneous Structure in Phonology." *Phonology* 10 (2): 281–306.

Brentari, Diane, Marie Coppola, Laura Mazzoni, and Susan Goldin-Meadow. 2012. "When Does a System Become Phonological? Handshape Production in Gesturers, Signers, and Homesigners." *Natural Language & Linguistic Theory* 30 (1): 1–31.

Briggs, Charles L. 2003. "Why Nation-States and Journalists Can't Teach People to Be Healthy: Power and Pragmatic Miscalculation in Public Discourses on Health." *Medical Anthropology Quarterly* 17 (3): 287–321.

Buffon, Georges-Louis Leclerc, comte de. 1801. *Histoire naturelle de Buffon*, vol. III. Edited by Pons-Joseph Bernard. Paris: Hacquart.

Central Bureau of Statistics. 2011. "National Population and Housing Census, 2011." Government of Nepal.

Cohen, Lawrence. 1998. *No Aging in India: Alzheimer's, the Bad Family, and Other Modern Things*. Oakland: University of California Press.

Coppola, Marie. 2002. "The Emergence of Grammatical Categories in Home Sign: Evidence from Family-Based Gesture Systems in Nicaragua." Ph.D. thesis, University of Rochester.

Cormier, Kearsy, David Quinto-Pozos, Zed Sevcikova, and Adam Schembri. 2012. "Lexicalisation and De-Lexicalisation Processes in Sign Languages: Comparing Depicting Constructions and Viewpoint Gestures." *Language & Communication* 32 (4): 329–48.

Coward, Harold. 1990. *Derrida and Indian Philosophy*. Albany: SUNY Press.

———. 1997. *The Sphoṭa Theory of Language*. Delhi: Motilal Banarsidass Publishers.

Crowe, Teresa Victoria, Bhuopendra Gimire, and Stephanie Trollo. 2016. "The Mental Health Needs of Deaf Adults in Nepal." *International Social Work* 59 (4): 508–22.

Das, Veena, and Renu Addlakha. 2001. "Disability and Domestic Citizenship: Voice, Gender, and the Making of the Subject." *Public Culture* 13 (3): 511–31.

Davis, Lennard J. 1995. *Enforcing Normalcy: Disability, Deafness, and the Body*. New York: Verso.

Debenport, Erin. 2013. "Continuous Perfectibility: Pueblo Propriety and the Consequences of Literacy." *Journal of Linguistic Anthropology* 22 (3): 201–19.

Debord, Guy. (1955) 2008. "Introduction to a Critique of Urban Geography." In *Critical Geographies: A Collection of Readings*, edited by Ken Knabb, 23–27. New York: Praxis (e)Press.

Defoe, Daniel. 1720. *The History of the Life and Adventures of Mr. Duncan Campbell, a Gentleman, Who Tho' Deaf And Dumb, Writes Down Any Stranger's Name at First Sight*. London: Nabu Press.

Deshpande, Madhav M. 1993. *Sanskrit & Prakrit: Sociolinguistic Issues*. Delhi: Motilal Banarsidass Publishers.

Desjarlais, Robert R. 2003. *Sensory Biographies: Lives and Deaths Among Nepal's Yolmo Buddhists*. Berkeley: University of California Press.

Dyssegaard, Birgit. 2000. "Emerging Educational Programs for Deaf Students in Mongolia and Nepal: A Special Report." In *The Deaf Child in the Family and at School: Essays in Honor of Kathryn P. Meadows-Orlans*, edited by Patricia Elizabeth Spencer, Carol J. Erting, and Marc Marschark, 239–54. Mahwah, NJ: Lawrence Erlbaum Associates.

Ebbinghaus, Horst, and Jens Hessmann. 1996. "Signs and Words: Accounting for Spoken Language Elements in German Sign Language." *International Review of Sign Linguistics* 1 (1): 23–56.

Eckert, Penelope. 2000. *Language Variation as Social Practice: The Linguistic Construction of Identity in Belten High*. New York: Wiley-Blackwell.

Farquhar, Judith. 2012. "Knowledge in Translation: Global Science, Local Things." In *Medicine and the Politics of Knowledge*, edited by Leslie Green and Susan Levine, 153–70. Cape Town: Human Sciences Research Council Press.

Frege, Gottlob. 1997. "On Sinn and Bedeutung." In *The Frege Reader*, edited by Michael Beaney, 151–70. New York: Wiley-Blackwell.

Friedner, Michele, and Jamie Osborne. 2013. "Audit Bodies: Embodied Participation, Disability Universalism, and Accessibility in India." *Antipode* 45 (1): 43–60.

Fusellier-Souza, Ivani. 2006. "Emergence and Development of Signed Languages: From a Semiogenetic Point of View." *Sign Language Studies* 7 (1): 30–56.

Gal, Susan, and Kathryn A. Woolard. 1995. "Constructing Languages and Publics: Authority and Representation." *Pragmatics* 5 (2): 129–38.

Ganeri, Jonardon. 1999. *Semantic Powers: Meaning and the Means of Knowing in Classical Indian Philosophy*. Oxford: Oxford University Press.

García Márquez, Gabriel. (1967) 2003. *One Hundred Years of Solitude*. Translated by Gregory Rabassa. New York: HarperCollins.

Garrett, Paul B. 2008. "Language Contact and Contact Languages." In *A Companion to Linguistic Anthropology*, edited by Alessandro Duranti, 46–72. Malden, MA: Blackwell.

Gell, Alfred. 1998. *Art and Agency: An Anthropological Theory*. Oxford: Oxford University Press.

Gellner, David N. 2007. *Resistance and the State: Nepalese Experiences.* New York: Berghahn Books.

Gerber, David A. 1990. "Listening to Disabled People: The Problem of Voice and Authority in Robert B. Edgerton's *The Cloak of Competence.*" *Disability, Handicap & Society* 5 (1): 3–23.

Giri, Ram Ashish. 2011. "Languages and Language Politics: How Invisible Language Politics Produces Visible Results in Nepal." *Language Problems & Language Planning* 35 (3): 197–221.

Goldin-Meadow, Susan. 2005a. *Hearing Gesture: How Our Hands Help Us Think.* Cambridge, MA: Harvard University Press.

———. 2005b. "Watching Language Grow." *Proceedings of the National Academy of Sciences of the United States of America* 102 (7): 2271–72.

Goodwin, Charles. 1994. "Professional Vision." *American Anthropologist* 96 (3): 606–33.

Graif, Peter. 2013. "Citing Signs: A Citational Model of Sign Language Phonology." Ph.D. thesis, CUNY Graduate Center.

Green, E. Mara. 2012. "'She's Saying What She Says': Interaction and Intelligibility in Deaf Nepal." Paper presented at the 2012 Annual Meeting of the American Anthropology Association, San Francisco, November 16.

———. 2014. "Natural Signs: Nepal's Deaf Society, Local Sign, and the Production of Communicative Sociality." Ph.D. thesis, University of California at Berkeley.

Greene, Paul. 2001. "Mixed Messages: Unsettled Cosmopolitanisms in Nepali Pop." *Popular Music* 20 (2): 169–87.

Grice, H. P. 1969. "Utterer's Meaning and Intention." *The Philosophical Review* 78 (2): 147–77.

Habermas, Jürgen. 1991. *The Structural Transformation of the Public Sphere: An Inquiry into a Category of Bourgeois Society.* Translated by Thomas Burger with Frederick Lawrence. Cambridge, MA: MIT Press.

Hahn, Harlan. 1997. "Advertising the Acceptably Employable Image." In *The Disability Studies Reader,* edited by Lennard J. Davis, 172–86. London: Routledge.

Hankins, Joseph. 2009. "Working through Skin: Making Leather, Making Multicultural Japan." Ph.D. thesis, University of Chicago.

Hansen, Nancy, and Chris Philo. 2007. "The Normality of Doing Things Differently: Bodies, Spaces and Disability Geography." *Tijdschrift voor Economische en Sociale Geografie* 98 (4): 493–506.

Hartford, Beverly. 2002. "Dangerous Words in a Strange Land: References to the Other in Nepalese Political Discourse." In *Surviving through Obliqueness: Language of Politics in Emerging Democracies*, edited by Samuel Gyasi Obeng and Beverly Hartford, 19–30. New York: Nova Publishers.

Harvey, David. 1989. *The Condition of Postmodernity: An Enquiry into the Origins of Cultural Change*. New York: Wiley-Blackwell.

Haualand, Hilde M. 2007. "The Two Week Village: The Significance of Sacred Occasions for the Deaf Community." In *Disability in Local and Global Worlds*, edited by Benedicte Ingstad and Susan Reynolds Whyte, 33–55. Oakland: University of California Press.

Helmreich, Stefan, and Michele Friedner. 2015. "Sound Studies Meets Deaf Studies." In *Sounding the Limits of Life: Essays in the Anthropology of Biology and Beyond*, by Stefan Helmreich, 164–72. Princeton, NJ: Princeton University Press.

Herder, Johann Gottfried. (1772) 2002. "Treatise on the Origin of Language." In *Herder: Philosophical Writings*, edited by Michael N. Forster, 65–166. Cambridge: Cambridge University Press.

Hindman, Heather. 2009. "Cosmopolitan Codifications: Elites, Expatriates, and Difference in Kathmandu, Nepal." *Identities: Global Studies in Culture and Power* 16 (3): 249–70.

Hockett, Charles F. 1960. "The Origin of Speech." *Scientific American* 203: 88–111.

Hoffmann, Erika G. 2008. "Standardization beyond Form: Ideologies, Institutions, and the Semiotics of Nepali Sign Language." Ph.D. thesis, University of Michigan.

Hoffmann-Dilloway, Erika G. 2008. "Metasemiotic Regimentation in the Standardization of Nepali Sign Language." *Journal of Linguistic Anthropology* 18 (2): 192–213.

———. 2011. "Lending a Hand: Competence through Cooperation in Nepal's Deaf Associations." *Language in Society* 40 (3): 285–306.

Holmberg, David H. 1996. *Order in Paradox: Myth, Ritual and Exchange among Nepal's Tamang*. Ithaca, NY: Cornell University Press.

Husserl, Edmund. 1960. *Cartesian Meditations: An Introduction to Phenomenology*. Translated by Dorion Cairns. The Hague: Nijhoff.

Ingstad, Benedicte, and Susan Reynolds Whyte. 2007. "Introduction: Disability Connections." In *Disability in Local and Global Worlds*, edited by Benedicte

Ingstad and Susan Reynolds Whyte, 1–29. Oakland: University of California Press.

Inoue, Miyako. 2004. "What Does Language Remember? Indexical Inversion and the Naturalized History of Japanese Women." *Journal of Linguistic Anthropology* 14 (1): 39–56.

Itard, Jean. 1842. *Les enfants sauvages*. Paris: Bibliothèque.

Jhala, Jayasinhji. 1997. "Speculations on the Concept of Indic Frontality Prompted by Questions on Portraiture." *Visual Anthropology* 10 (1): 49–66.

Johnson, Andrew Alan. 2013. "Progress and Its Ruins: Ghosts, Migrants, and the Uncanny in Thailand." *Cultural Anthropology* 28 (2): 299–319.

Johnson, Russell J., and Jane E. Johnson. 2016. "Distinction between West Bengal Sign Language and Indian Sign Language Based on Statistical Assessment." *Sign Language Studies* 16 (4): 473–99.

Justice, Judith. 1989. *Plans, Policies, and People: Foreign Aid and Health Development*. Berkeley: University of California Press.

Kelly, John D. 1996. "What was Sanskrit for? Metadiscursive Strategies in Ancient India." In *Ideology and Status of Sanskrit*, edited by Jan E. M. Houben, 87–108. Leiden: Brill Academic Publishers.

Kendon, Adam. 1980. "A Description of a Deaf-Mute Sign Language from the Enga Province of Papua New Guinea with Some Comparative Discussion." *Semiotica* 31 (1–2): 1–34.

———. 2004. *Gesture: Visible Action as Utterance*. Cambridge: Cambridge University Press.

Khanal, Upendra. 2013. "Age-Related Sociolinguistic Variation in Sign Languages, with Particular Reference to Nepali Sign." *Nepalese Linguistics* 28: 64–70.

Kimmel, Michael. 2008. "Properties of Cultural Embodiment: Lessons from the Anthropology of the Body." In *Body, Language, and Mind*, vol. 2: *Sociocultural Situatedness*, edited by Roslyn M. Frank, René Dirven, Tom Ziemke, and Enrique Bernárdez, 77–108. Berlin: Mouton de Gruyter.

Klima, Edward S., and Ursula Bellugi. 1979. *The Signs of Language*. Cambridge, MA: Harvard University Press.

Kripke, Saul A. 1980. *Naming and Necessity*. Cambridge, MA: Harvard University Press.

Kunreuther, Laura. 2006. "Technologies of the Voice: FM Radio, Telephone, and the Nepali Diaspora in Kathmandu." *Cultural Anthropology* 21 (3): 323–53.

———. 2009. "Between Love and Property: Voice, Sentiment, and Subjectivity in the Reform of Daughter's Inheritance in Nepal." *American Ethnologist* 36 (3): 545–62.

Ladd, Paddy. 2003. *Understanding Deaf Culture: In Search of Deafhood.* Bristol, UK: Multilingual Matters.

Lakoff, George. 1990. *Women, Fire, and Dangerous Things: What Categories Reveal about the Mind.* Chicago: University of Chicago Press.

Landstreicher, Wolfi. 2002. *From Politics to Life: Ridding Anarchy of the Leftist Millstone.* Portland, OR: Venomous Butterfly Publications.

Lane, Harlan L. 2010. *When the Mind Hears: A History of the Deaf.* New York: Random House.

Lane, Harlan L., Robert Hoffmeister, and Benjamin J. Bahan. 1996. *A Journey into the Deaf-World.* San Diego, CA: Dawn Sign Press.

Latour, Bruno, and Steve Woolgar. 1986. *Laboratory Life: The Construction of Scientific Facts.* Princeton, NJ: Princeton University Press.

Lawoti, Mahendra. 2005. *Towards a Democratic Nepal: Inclusive Political Institutions for a Multicultural Society.* London: Sage.

Lewis, David. 2001. *On the Plurality of Worlds.* New York: Wiley.

Lewis, M. Paul., Gary F. Simons, and Charles D. Fennig, eds. 2013. *Ethnologue: Languages of the World.* Dallas, TX: SIL International.

Liddell, Scott K. 2003. *Grammar, Gesture, and Meaning in American Sign Language.* Cambridge: Cambridge University Press.

Liechty, Mark. 2003. *Suitably Modern: Making Middle-Class Culture in a New Consumer Society.* Princeton, NJ: Princeton University Press.

Little, Paul, Alison Bridges, Rajendra Guragain, Del Friedman, Rakesh Prasad, and Neil Weir. 1993. "Hearing Impairment and Ear Pathology in Nepal." *The Journal of Laryngology & Otology* 107 (5): 395–400.

Lucas, Ceil, and Clayton Valli. 1992. *Language Contact in the American Deaf Community.* Bingley, UK: Emerald Group Publishing.

Macpherson, Hannah. 2010. "Non-Representational Approaches to Body–Landscape Relations." *Geography Compass* 4 (1): 1–13.

Manning, Paul. 2012. *Semiotics of Drink and Drinking.* New York: Continuum.

Maskarinec, Gregory G. 1995. *The Rulings of the Night: An Ethnography of Nepalese Shaman Oral Texts.* Madison: University of Wisconsin Press.

Matilal, Bimal Krishna. 1998. *The Character of Logic in India.* Albany: SUNY Press.

Mayberry, Rachel I., and Ellen B. Eichen. 1991. "The Long-Lasting Advantage of Learning Sign Language in Childhood: Another Look at the Critical Period for Language Acquisition." *Journal of Memory and Language* 30 (4): 486–512.

McNeill, David. 2005. *Gesture and Thought*. Chicago: University of Chicago Press.

Meier, Richard P. 1991. "Language Acquisition by Deaf Children." *American Scientist* 79 (1): 60–70.

Miles, Michael. 2001. "Studying Responses to Disability in South Asian Histories: Approaches Personal, Prakrital and Pragmatical." *Disability & Society* 16 (1): 143–60.

Mitchell, Ross E. 2005. "How Many Deaf People Are There in the United States? Estimates from the Survey of Income and Program Participation." *Journal of Deaf Studies and Deaf Education* 11 (1): 112–19.

Monaghan, Leila, Constanze Schmaling, Karen Nakamura, and Graham H. Turner, eds. 2003. *Many Ways to Be Deaf: International Variation in Deaf Communities*. Washington, DC: Gallaudet University Press.

Morford, Jill P. 2002. "The Expression of Motion Events in Homesign." *Sign Language & Linguistics* 5 (1): 55–71.

Morford, Jill P., and Susan Goldin-Meadow. 1997. "From Here and Now to There and Then: The Development of Displaced Reference in Homesign and English." *Child Development* 68 (3): 420–35.

Nakassis, Constantine V. 2013. "Brands and Their Surfeits." *Cultural Anthropology* 28 (1): 111–26.

Nepali Sign Language National Development Committee. 2003. *Nepali Sign Language Dictionary*. Kathmandu: Nepal National Federation of the Deaf and Hard of Hearing.

Ochs, Elinor, and Merav Shohet. 2006. "The Cultural Structuring of Mealtime Socialization." *New Directions for Child and Adolescent Development* 111: 35–49.

Okrent, Arika. 2012. "Why Great Sign Language Interpreters Are So Animated." *The Atlantic*, November. 2.

Onta, Pratyoush Raj. 2006. *Mass Media in post-1990 Nepal*. Kathmandu: Martin Chautari.

Padden, Carol, and Tom Humphries. 1989. *Deaf in America: Voices from a Culture*. Cambridge, MA: Harvard University Press.

———. 2009. *Inside Deaf Culture*. Cambridge, MA: Harvard University Press.

Pant, Mohan, and Shuji Funo. 2003. "Considerations on the Layout Pattern of Streets and Settlement Blocks of Thimi: A Study on the Planning Modules of Kathmandu Valley Towns (Part I)." *Journal of Architecture, Planning, and Environmental Engineering* 574: 83–90.

Paterson, Kevin, and Bill Hughes. 1999. "Disability Studies and Phenomenology: The Carnal Politics of Everyday Life." *Disability & Society* 14 (5): 597–610.

Patton, Laurie L. 2011. *Bringing the Gods to Mind: Mantra and Ritual in Early Indian Sacrifice.* Berkeley: University of California Press.

Paudel, Ram Chandra. 2010. "An Appraisal on the Origin of the Veda." *Bodhi: An Interdisciplinary Journal* 3 (1): 120–24.

Perniss, Pamela. 2007. "Space and Iconicity in German Sign Language (DGS)." Ph.D. thesis, Radboud University Nijmegen.

Pigg, Stacy Leigh. 1992. "Investing Social Categories through Place: Social Representations and Development in Nepal." *Comparative Studies in Society and History* 34 (3): 491–513.

———. 1996. "The Credible and the Credulous: The Question of 'Villagers' Beliefs' in Nepal." *Cultural Anthropology* 11 (2): 160–201.

———. 2001. "Languages of Sex and AIDS in Nepal: Notes on the Social Production of Commensurability." *Cultural Anthropology* 16 (4): 481–541.

Plato. 2008. *Cratylus.* Translated by Benjamin Jowett. New York: Arc Manor LLC.

Pollock, Sheldon. 2006. *The Language of the Gods in the World of Men: Sanskrit, Culture, and Power in Premodern India.* Berkeley: University of California Press.

Prasad, Lakshman. 2003. *Status of People with Disability in Nepal.* Kathmandu: Rajesh Prasad Shrivastav.

Quine, Willard van Orman. 1960. *Word and Object.* Cambridge, MA: MIT Press.

Quinto-Pozos, David. 2007. "Can Constructed Action Be Considered Obligatory?" *Lingua* 117 (7): 1285–314.

———. 2010. "Register Variation in Mimetic Gestural Complements to Signed Language." *Journal of Pragmatics* 42 (3): 557–84.

Rapp, Rayna, and Faye Ginsburg. 2011. "Reverberations: Disability and the New Kinship Imaginary." *Anthropological Quarterly* 84 (2): 379–410.

Rath, Gayatri. 2000. *Linguistic Philosophy in Vakyapadiya.* Delhi: Bharatiya Vidya Prakashan.

Rée, Jonathan. 1999. *I See a Voice: Deafness, Language, and the Senses*. London: Metropolitan Books.

Robbins, Joel. 2001. "Ritual Communication and Linguistic Ideology: A Reading and Partial Reformulation of Rappaport's Theory of Ritual." *Current Anthropology* 42 (5): 591–614.

———. 2008. "On Not Knowing Other Minds: Confession, Intention, and Linguistic Exchange in a Papua New Guinea Community." *Anthropological Quarterly* 81 (2): 421–29.

Robbins, Joel, and Alan Rumsey. 2008. "Cultural and Linguistic Anthropology and the Opacity of Other Minds." *Anthropology Quarterly* 81 (2): 407–20.

Rosenstock, Rachel. 2008. "The Role of Iconicity in International Sign." *Sign Language Studies* 8 (2): 131–59.

Rosenthal, Abigail. 2009. "Lost in Transcription: The Problematics of Commensurability in Academic Representations of American Sign Language." *Text & Talk: An Interdisciplinary Journal of Language* 29 (5): 595–614.

Russell, Marta. 2002. "What Disability Civil Rights Cannot Do: Employment and Political Economy." *Disability & Society* 17 (2): 117–35.

Sacks, Oliver W. 1989. *Seeing Voices: A Journey into the Land of the Deaf*. Berkeley: University of California Press.

Sadler, Simon. 1999. *The Situationist City*. Cambridge, MA: MIT Press.

Sandler, Wendy. 1989. *Phonological Representation of the Sign: Linearity and Nonlinearity in American Sign Language*. Berlin: Walter de Gruyter.

———. 2008. "A Sonority Cycle in American Sign Language." *Phonology* 10 (2): 243–79.

Sandler, Wendy, Mark Aronoff, Irit Meir, and Carol A. Padden. 2011. "The Gradual Emergence of Phonological Form in a New Language." *Natural Language & Linguistic Theory* 29 (2): 1–41.

Sandler, Wendy, Irit Meir, Carol A. Padden, Mark Aronoff, and Jeremy Sabloff. 2005. "The Emergence of Grammar: Systematic Structure in a New Language." *Proceedings of the National Academy of Sciences of the United States of America* 102 (7): 2661–65.

Sapir, Edward. 1921. *Language*. Cambridge: Cambridge University Press.

———. (1938) 2001. "Why Cultural Anthropology Needs the Psychiatrist." *Psychiatry: Interpersonal and Biological Processes* 64 (1): 2–10.

Senghas, Ann. 2003. "Intergenerational Influence and Ontogenetic Development in the Emergence of Spatial Grammar in Nicaraguan Sign Language." *Cognitive Development* 18 (4): 511–31.

————. 2004. "Children Creating Core Properties of Language: Evidence from an Emerging Sign Language in Nicaragua." *Science* 305 (5691): 1779–82.

————. 2005. "Language Emergence: Clues from a New Bedouin Sign." *Current Biology* 15 (12): R463–65.

Senghas, Ann, and Marie Coppola. 2001. "Children Creating Language: How Nicaraguan Sign Language Acquired a Spatial Grammar." *Psychological Science* 12 (4): 323–28.

Sharp, Keith, and Sarah Earle. 2002. "Feminism, Abortion and Disability: Irreconcilable Differences?" *Disability & Society* 17 (2): 137–45.

Shneiderman, Sara. 2014. "Reframing Ethnicity: Academic Tropes, Recognition beyond Politics, and Ritualized Action between Nepal and India." *American Anthropologist* 116 (2): 279–95.

Shrestha, Nanda R. 1997. *In the Name of Development: A Reflection on Nepal.* Lanham, MD: University Press of America.

Shuttleworth, R. P. 2004. "Stigma, Community, Ethnography: Joan Ablon's Contribution to the Anthropology of Impairment-Disability." *Medical Anthropology Quarterly* 18 (2): 139–61.

Sibscota, George. 1670. *The Deaf and Dumb Man's Discourse.* London: Scolar.

Sider, Theodore. 2003. *Four-Dimensionalism: An Ontology of Persistence and Time.* Oxford: Clarendon Press.

Slusser, Mary S. 1982. *Nepal Mandala: A Cultural Study of the Kathmandu Valley.* Princeton, NJ: Princeton University Press.

Smith, Brian K. 1986. "Ritual, Knowledge, and Being: Initiation and Veda Study in Ancient India." *Numen* 33 (1): 65–89.

Sonntag, Selma K. 1995. "Ethnolinguistic Identity and Language Policy in Nepal." *Nationalism and Ethnic Politics* 1 (4): 108–20.

Sparrow, Robert. 2005. "Defending Deaf Culture: The Case of Cochlear Implants." *Journal of Political Philosophy* 13 (2): 135–52.

Spivak, Gayatri Chakrovarty. 1988. "Can the Subaltern Speak?" In *Marxism and the Interpretation of Culture*, edited by Cary Nelson and Lawrence Grossberg, 271–316. Urbana: University of Illinois Press.

Stallybrass, Peter, and Allon White. 1986. *The Politics and Poetics of Transgression.* Ithaca, NY: Cornell University Press.

————. 2007. "The City: The Sewer, the Gaze, and the Contaminating Touch." In *Beyond the Body Proper*, edited by Margaret Lock and Judith Farquhar, 266–85. Durham, NC: Duke University Press.

Stokoe, William C. 1960. "Sign Language Structure: An Outline of the Visual Communication Systems of the American Deaf." *Studies in Linguistics: Occasional Papers* 8.

Stokoe, William C., Dorothy C. Casterline, and Carl G. Croneberg. 1976. *A Dictionary of American Sign Language on Linguistic Principles*. Burtonsville, MD: Linstok Press.

Strathern, Marilyn. 1988. *The Gender of the Gift: Problems with Women and Problems with Society in Melanesia*. Oakland: University of California Press.

———. 2011. "What is a Parent?" *HAU: Journal of Ethnographic Theory* 1 (1): 245–78.

Susman, Joan. 1994. "Disability, Stigma and Deviance." *Social Science & Medicine* 38 (1): 15–22.

Sutton, Valerie. 1995. *Lessons in Sign Writing*. La Jolla, CA: The Deaf Action Committee for SignWriting.

Swinbourne, Charlie. 2015. "The Question: Could You Spot a Deaf Person in a Crowded Room? And Is There Such a Thing as a 'Deafdar'? (BSL)." The Limping Chicken, February 14. http://limpingchicken.com/2015/02/14/the-question-could-you-spot-a-deaf-person-in-a-crowded-room-and-is-there-such-a-thing-as-a-deafdar-bsl/.

Taub, Sarah F. 2001. *Language from the Body: Iconicity and Metaphor in American Sign Language*. Cambridge: Cambridge University Press.

Torigoe, Takashi, and Wataru Takei. 2002. "A Descriptive Analysis of Pointing and Oral Movements in a Home Sign System." *Sign Language Studies* 2 (3): 281–95.

Turin, Mark. 2004. "Minority Language Politics in Nepal and the Himalayas." Paper presented for Scalla 2004 Working Conference "Crossing the Digital Divide: Shaping Technologies to Meet Human Needs," Kathmandu, Nepal, January 5–7. https://pdfs.semanticscholar.org/1215/1246f36442c0425f444ed1dd92c4b6cd26b8.pdf.

Turner, Ralph L. 1990. *A Comparative and Etymological Dictionary of the Nepali Language*. London: K. Paul, Trench, Trubner.

Voeltz, F. K. Erhard, and Christa Kilian-Hatz, eds. 2001. *Ideophones*. Amsterdam: John Benjamins Publishing Company.

Vološinov, V. N. (1929) 1986. *Marxism and the Philosophy of Language*. Translated by Ladislav Matejka and I. R. Titunik. Cambridge, MA: Harvard University Press.

Warner, Michael. 1990. *The Letters of the Republic: Publication and the Public Sphere in Eighteenth-Century America.* Cambridge, MA: Harvard University Press.

———. 1993. "The Mass Public and the Mass Subject." In *American Literary Studies: A Methodological Reader,* edited by Michael A. Elliott and Claudia Stokes, 243–63. New York: NYU Press.

———. 2002. "Publics and Counterpublics." *Public Culture* 14 (1): 49–90.

Whelpton, John. 2012. "Political Identity in Nepal: State, Nation, and Community." In *Nationalism and Ethnicity in a Hindu Kingdom: The Politics of Culture in Contemporary Nepal,* edited by David N. Gellner, Joanna Pfaff-Czarnecka, and John Whelpton, 39–78. London: Routledge.

Whitehead, Harry. 2010. "The Agency of Yearning on the Northwest Coast of Canada: Franz Boas, George Hunt and the Salvage of Autochthonous Culture." *Memory Studies* 3 (3): 215–23.

Wickenden, Mary. 2011. "Whose Voice is That? Issues of Identity, Voice and Representation Arising in an Ethnographic Study of the Lives of Disabled Teenagers Who Use Augmentative and Alternative Communication (AAC)." *Disability Studies Quarterly* 31 (4). http://dsq-sds.org/article/view/1724/1772.

Wilke, Annette, and Oliver Moebus. 2011. *Sound and Communication: An Aesthetic Cultural History of Sanskrit Hinduism.* Berlin: Walter de Gruyter.

Williams, Bronwyn. 2012. "The World on Your Screen: New Media, Remix, and the Politics of Cross-Cultural Contact." In *New Media Literacies and Participatory Popular Culture across Borders,* edited by Bronwyn Williams and Amy A. A. Zenger, 17–32. New York: Routledge.

World Health Organization. 2011. "World Report on Disability." http://www.who.int/disabilities/world_report/2011/report.pdf.

Yadava, Yogendra P. 2007. "Linguistic Diversity in Nepal: Perspectives on Language Policy." Paper presented at an international seminar on "Constitutionalism and Diversity in Nepal," Tribhuvan University, Kathmandu, August 22–24. http://www.uni-biclcfeld.de/midea/pdf/Yogendra.pdf.

Yelle, Robert A. 2003. *Explaining Mantras: Ritual, Rhetoric, and the Dream of a Natural Language in Hindu Tantra.* New York: Psychology Press.

Acknowledgments

The central claim of this book is that things are present or absent in context by virtue of the histories of perception that surround them. The text I have presented here is no exception. It is the consequence of many debts accumulated in the course of its own creation, though few of these debts are readily visible here in its most tangible, permanent, and public form. In this section (far too short), I hope to make some of those histories more intelligible.

Throughout my research and writing, I was supported by a number of different programs. These include the Amherst College Donald S. Pitkin Fellowship in Anthropology, the University of Chicago Century Fellowship, two Foreign Language and Area Studies (FLAS) fellowships in Kathmandu, the Fulbright-Hays Doctoral Dissertation Research Abroad Grant, a grant from the Endangered Language Initiative at the CUNY Graduate Center, and ongoing financial support from the Open Institute for Social Science in Kathmandu. On the other side of fieldwork, I owe a great deal to my editors at Hau for their dedication to this project from its earlier, much rougher forms, and especially to my anonymous readers, whose deep insight and meticulous attention I've done my best to honor.

I have also benefited from a number of unusually generous mentors. Deborah Gewertz was the first to teach me anthropology, and, though her influence precedes this project, it is consequential throughout. Drucilla Ronchen taught me more about fieldwork in deaf communities than I think I'll ever fully realize. The members of my dissertation committee, Juliette Blevins, John Kelly, and

Michael Silverstein, are all deeply present in the pages of this volume. I am grateful for their time, teaching, and support. I am especially grateful to my committee chair, Judith Farquhar, who has been a mentor in the truest and broadest sense of the word. Thank you.

Grad school was better because Abigail Rosenthal was there, too. Her clarity and generosity through countless early drafts propelled this book forward. Gretchen Pfeil has been a wonderful collaborator and a true friend. Amanda Snellinger knows how to get anything done in Kathmandu, and I have learned a lot from her. Sanjib Pokhrel was there from the absolute beginning, and his friendship and teaching provide the foundation to a great deal here. Surendra, Sayuja, Ayushman, and Prastut Shrestha gave me a home and taught me how to be a person in Nepal, and for that I will always be grateful. There are few people in this world with as much insight and resolve as Dhirendra Nalbo, and his patient attention has improved this book in countless ways. Frank Bechter's influence on this work is singular. I have no idea what he must have thought when I sent him that naïve if wildly enthusiastic email all those years ago, but I couldn't have asked for a better friend and mentor. Mara Green is present in perhaps every page of this book, in insights gleaned from the thousand subtle, insightful, impassioned, critical, generous, and often challenging conversations I had with her. As our mutual acquaintances in deaf Nepal are always very happy to remind me, she remains the better signer. I will always be grateful for her friendship.

Above all else, this work has been possible only because a great many deaf people in Kathmandu invited me into their lives. To name just a few, my sincere thanks go to Kiran Acharya, Rashmi Amatya, Bikash Dangol, Nagendra Gurung, Raghav Bir Joshi, Sushil Karmacharya, Sitaram Karnal, Uttam Maharjan, Deepak Shakya, Dipawali Sharma, Rojina Shrestha, Sachin Shrestha, Sanobhai Timilsina, and Satyadevi Wagle. The insight, dedication, kindness, and boundless humor you shared with me were more than I ever deserved. I only hope those things are reflected in these pages.

I am grateful to my family—Theresa Graif, Michael Graif, Benjamin Graif, Joseph Graif, Patricia Martin, Richard Martin, and especially Linda Atwood—for being always ready at hand with their support. Mateo and Soren were wonderful writing companions, and they always gave me a reason to look forward to coming home. Though all flaws of analysis in this book remain my own, any typos that exist might be traced back to the two of them, enthusiastic as they were from an early age to help me write. Most of all, and with all of my love, I am grateful to Sonya. This book is dedicated to her.

Index

A

absence, (see presence and absence)
absurdity, 42, 43, 73, 173
activism, 32, 47, 51, 52, 108–110, 119–121, 124–129
anthropology of the deaf, 51–52, 74–75, 122, 135, 190
arbitrariness, (see iconicity and arbitrariness)
Arjun, 1–36, 37–38, 41–42, 45–46, 66, 93, 189
Arjun's notebooks, 5, 9, 15, 24–26, 33–36, 42, 45, 189
asymmetries
    as a basis of radical difference, 135, 190
    of experience, 46, 50, 66, 70, 74, 133, 134, 173
    of linguistic function, 22, 94, 116, 153
attention
    and ethnography, 9, 47, 136, 153
    as radical praxis, 34–36, 45, 129, 173, 189–190
    hearing habits of, 38, 44, 67–68, 69, 94
    techniques of, 48–50, 78, 102, 105, 160, 162
authenticity, 2, 26, 48, 91, 162, 176
awareness
    dialogic nature of, 46
    discourses of, 32, 64, 70, 138, 180
    of objects, 45, 135

B

bahira (deaf), 62–64
Bakery Cafe, 163–169
Bechter, Frank, 43, 128, 166
being
    and perceiving, 74–75
    and becoming, 69, 179, 185–186
    deaf ways of, 52, 136, 183, 187–190
    in social place, 51, 66
    in South Asian philosophy, 158, 184–186
blindness, 13–14, 39–42, 75, 77
brahman (absolute), 158–159
braille, 39–45, 77

C

category

and instance, 32, 56, 66
as basis of encounter, 43, 52,
　63–64, 121, 169, 174
in ethnography, 35, 135
material conditions of, 54, 138
citation, 84, 96, 125, 159–162, 167–169
convert culture, 43, 128, 166
cultural difference
　and identity, 7–8, 89, 95, 136
　and other minds, 6, 111
　constitution in context, 135
　effacement of, 70–71, 122, 190
　stakes of, 90, 93
　substance of, 34–36, 42, 47, 54, 122,
　　132
　seeing, 41, 52, 69, 190, 193
　value of, 7, 52, 58, 136

D

deaf/Deaf distinctions, 52
deafdar, 48
deaf studies, 7, 50
deaf worlds
　and hearing things, 36, 133, 126,
　　166
　as architecture of perception,
　　48–53, 102, 125, 134–135, 162,
　　168
　community, 2, 16, 20, 50, 58, 68,
　　83, 90, 96, 104, 121, 126–129,
　　161
　culture, 38, 52, 122, 128, 166, 193
　deafness of, 52–53, 69
　geography of, 47, 51–61
　hearing knowledge of, 7, 42, 50,
　　86, 173
　kinship, 4, 33, 60, 83, 110, 119–121,
　　133, 188
　teaching the hearing to see,
　　44–46, 119, 134–135
deixis, 55, 80, 182
desire, 3, 9, 34, 187

Desjarlais, Robert, 121, 186
development rhetoric, 3, 26, 42, 55–56,
　64, 109, 113
dharma (law), 92
dialectic, 178, 185–188
dictionaries
　as ideological projects, 5, 65,
　　96–104, 148, 151, 164–168
　as sites of experience, 35–36,
　　37–38, 85, 97–99, 189
disability, 7, 14, 23, 43–44, 47, 48, 69,
　122, 126
disability studies, 54
displacement, 29, 31, 95, 111, 113, 121,
　134, 185
duality of patterning, 137–139

E

echoes, 79, 123, 158–162, 187
efficacy, 8–9, 15, 24, 29, 31, 37–38, 91,
　139, 155–157
embodiment, 31, 45, 80–81, 102
empty space
　impulse to fill, 8, 31
　in things and people, 24–25,
　　29–31, 108
　productivity of, 12, 68, 130
entanglement, 7, 24, 31, 34–36, 46,
　66–67, 93, 96, 175
ethnographic theory, 15, 23, 25, 36, 45,
　51, 102, 134–136, 189–190
exceptions (see typicality and
　exception)
exemplification (see typicality and
　exception)

F

fakes (see real and fake)
foreground and background, 34–36,
　38, 44–45, 48–49, 80, 100, 125,
　190

G

gesture, 8, 20–23, 48–49, 71–72, 79,
    102, 141–144, 164–166, 168
grammar, 16, 20–23, 64–65, 95, 102,
    140

H

habituation, 15, 23, 34–35, 105, 137–138,
    194
hearing, the feeling of being, 66–67,
    118
hearing worlds
    and deaf things, 40, 50–51, 66, 119,
        126, 133
    as architecture of perception, 9,
        25, 29–32, 36, 38, 47–50, 61–68,
        74, 118, 173–175, 184–190
    deaf knowledge of, 34, 38, 41,
        50–51, 94, 122–124, 133
Heidegger, Martin, 45
homesign, 19–22, 84, 112, 142

I

iconicity and arbitrariness, 17, 80,
    137–141, 149–152, 162, 167–168
intelligibility
    asymmetries of, 69–74, 84, 88, 131,
        138, 151, 153, 173
    conditions of, 51–53, 60, 85, 94–95,
        104, 122, 131, 140, 189–190
    management of, 95, 103, 105,
        113–119, 123–125, 128, 133, 148,
        162, 167–168
    theory of, 44–45, 75, 80, 105, 133,
        187, 193
intersubjectivity, 6, 45, 80, 140, 164,
    166, 174, 185, 180
isolation, 2, 13, 30, 38, 40, 46, 54,
    108–109, 120, 124, 125

J

Joshi, Raghav Bir, 68–74, 104, 119, 142,
    189

K

KAD (Kathmandu Association of
    the Deaf), 38, 42–43, 53, 56–59, 68,
    78, 124–129
Keller, Helen, 12
kurā (talk/thing/idea), 186–188

L

landscape and architecture, 51, 55–56,
    60, 122–123, 126–129, 138, 173, 181,
    191
language
    as accumulated history, 77–85, 104,
        162, 155–169
    as community, 2, 13, 54–55, 89, 109,
        120–121, 161
    as competency, 16–17, 35, 53, 65, 79,
        82, 97, 137–141, 167
    as difference, 19–22, 34, 38–39, 44,
        86–93
    as human capacity, 40–41, 142–143
    as object of notice, 49–50, 96,
        111–133
    as perceptual attunement, 84–85,
        94–96, 102–105, 168
    as presentation of self, 23, 95,
        117–118, 140, 152–154, 157–158
    as purposeful action, 31, 77–85,
        102, 117, 137, 149, 155
lāṭo (dumb, mute), 14, 40, 62–64, 114,
    121, 172–175
lorem ipsum, 129–136

M

Mahesh, 77–85, 100, 104, 166

Matilal, Bimal Krishna, 184, 187
meaning
    and being, 30–32, 166
    and form, 34, 129, 138
    and meaninglessness, 115, 118, 138
    as a historical process, 22, 24,
        83–85
    as a social act, 80, 96
    as way to fill gaps, 8, 66, 152
    being forced to experience,
        130–131
    deaf theories of, 79, 131, 152–153,
        160–162
    tacit expectation of, 16–17, 153
misrecognition, 9, 28, 40, 42, 173
mother languages, 120–121
mutual expectancy, 80, 162
mutually-aligned perception, 23, 25,
    47, 104–105, 108, 166, 187

N

nakalī (counterfeit, duplicate), 26, 35
names, 53, 55–56, 60, 77–85, 104–105, 149
natural signs, 16–17, 20, 91, 99, 114, 119
Naxal School for the Deaf, 58, 68, 107
NFDH (Nepal National Federation
    of the Deaf and Hard of Hear-
    ing), 57, 68–70
NSL (see signed language)

O

objecthood, 29, 135, 168, 187
ontology, 29, 44–46, 141, 155, 166,
    184–185, 187
opacity (see transparency and opacity)
other minds problem, 6, 9, 11–12, 26,
    85

P

pantomime, 8, 16, 21–22, 72, 139–141

perception and non-perception:
    of agency, 6, 10–11, 25, 31, 35–36,
        88, 91
    of interiority, 7–9, 15, 25, 33, 88,
        108, 118, 184
    of language, 19, 22, 96, 139, 153
    of social history, 17, 20–23, 26, 29,
        96, 128, 153, 132, 162
perdurance, 11, 71, 167, 184–188
perfect signs, 154–155, 158–159
personhood, 15, 40–41, 69, 175, 181–187
phenomenology, 35, 45, 75, 101–102,
    158, 164, 173–175, 183
pidgins, 20, 72, 84
prakṛtik (natural), 91–93, 156
pranks, 48–50, 131, 173
presence and absence
    as echoes, 158, 162, 187
    of social facts, 6, 29, 31–32, 59–60,
        63, 66, 105, 119
    sensitivity to, 50, 53, 67–68, 75, 80,
        96, 130, 173
    theory of, 25, 45, 92, 157–158,
        182–190
properties of objects, 26, 29, 175,
    184–189
prosthesis, 22, 58, 83, 124

R

radical theory, 36, 135–136, 190
real and fake, 26–29, 93, 131
reference, 16, 42, 53–55, 79–85, 94–95,
    101–104, 147–151, 158, 164–169, 174,
    181–186

S

salience, 22, 45, 51, 80, 85, 94, 102, 134,
    164, 184
semantic slippage, 63, 120, 184, 188
sense, 24–25, 29–32, 34–36, 37–38, 45,
    118, 129, 133, 189

signed language
  and spoken language, 20, 40, 68,
    139
  boundaries of, 19–22, 100–105, 153
  demographics of, 13, 54–55, 78, 85,
    96, 100, 108, 120–121, 126, 167
  hearing encounters with, 16–23,
    49–50, 71–72, 87–88, 95, 112,
    140, 172
  history of, 58, 141–143, 166–167
  linguistic study of, 19–22, 139–141
  NSL Development Committee,
    156, 162, 171
  "short" and "long", 143–151, 165
  standardization, 96–100, 144,
    152–154, 159, 162, 168
  structure of, 17, 64, 97, 100,
    104–105, 141, 159, 166–167
  teaching, 38, 97, 107–110, 152, 160
  variation, 82–83, 91, 100–105,
    141–151
sojho (simple), 30, 87–88, 93
sphoṭa (linguistic theory), 31
stigma, 4, 46, 88, 122

T

tacit knowledge, 44, 91, 108
talk/intelligible, 190
Thirbam Sadak, 55–61, 119, 122–124,
  171
Tito Satya (television program), 26
transparency and opacity

burden of, 23, 34–35, 68, 88, 94
experience of, 9, 15, 21–22, 32, 92,
  95, 99, 113–114, 139
strategic management of, 34,
  113–119, 118, 133, 152–161
typicality and exception, 7, 12–13, 32,
  40, 53, 60, 74, 88, 166

U

universe, nature of, 92, 155
urban/rural divides, 2, 46, 89, 107–119,
  133–34

V

vectors of citation, (see citation)
Vedas, 155–159, 162, 166
virtuosity, 32, 35, 49, 116, 133, 166, 183,
  187
voice, 13, 63, 69, 95, 105–107, 113, 120,
  126–127, 147, 173

W

words
  and things, 80, 102, 150, 155, 162
  inertia of, 173
  limits of, 101–103

Y

yo and *tyo* (this and that), 181

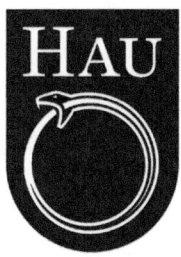

HAU Books is committed to publishing the most distinguished texts in classic and advanced anthropological theory. The titles aim to situate ethnography as the prime heuristic of anthropology, and return it to the forefront of conceptual developments in the discipline. HAU Books is sponsored by some of the world's most distinguished anthropology departments and research institutions, and releases its titles in both print editions and open-access formats.

www.haubooks.com

Supported by
Hau-N. E. T.
Network of Ethnographic Theory

University of Aarhus – EPICENTER (DK)
University of Amsterdam (NL)
Australian National University – Library (AU)
University of Bergen (NO)
Brown University (US)
California Institute of Integral Studies (US)
University of Campinas (BR)
University of Canterbury (NZ)
University College London (UK)
University of Cologne – The Global South Studies Centre (DE)
and City Library of Cologne (DE)
University of Colorado Boulder Libraries (US)
Cornell University (US)
University of Edinburgh (UK)
The Graduate Institute – Geneva Library (CH)
University of Groningen (NL)
Harvard University (US)
The Higher School of Economics in St. Petersburg (RU)
Humboldt University of Berlin (DE)
Indiana University Library (US)
Johns Hopkins University (US)
University of Kent (UK)
Lafayette College Library (US)
London School of Economics and Political Science (UK)
Institute of Social Sciences of the University of Lisbon (PL)
Ludwig Maximilian University of Munich (DE)
University of Manchester (UK)
The University of Manchester Library (UK)
Max-Planck Institute for the Study of Religious and Ethnic
Diversity at Göttingen (DE)
Musée de Quai Branly (FR)
Museu Nacional – UFRJ (BR)
Norwegian Museum of Cultural History (NO)
University of Oslo (NO)
University of Oslo Library (NO)
Princeton University (US)
University of Rochester (US)
SOAS, University of London (UK)
University of Sydney (AU)
University of Toronto Libraries (CA)

www.haujournal.org/haunet